Intermittent Fasting for Women Over 50

A Guide that Explains the Pros and Cons of Intermittent Fasting

Author

Rachel R. Jones

Table of Contents

Chapter 5: Types of Intermittent Fasting

Chapter 6: The 5:2 diet

Chapter 7: Fundamentals of Intermittent Fasting

Chapter 8: Fasting- Tips & Tricks for Woman

Chapter 9: The Benefits and Drawbacks to Exercising Whilst On a Fast

Chapter 10: Learning What Is Wrong and How to Make It Right!

Chapter 11: OMAD Diet

Chapter 12: 10 Popular Mistakes to Avoid During Intermittent Fasting

Conclusion

Introduction

Intermittent fasting is an eating practice under which you alternate between eating and fasting times. "Intermittent fasting may be part of a healthier lifestyle," according to Johns Hopkins which Medicine neuroscientist, Ph.D., who has researched the health effects of intermittent fasting over 25 years and embraced it himself around 20 years ago. According to him, evidence shows that reducing one "eating time" will help you live longer and reduce the risk of chronic diseases.

Do you think you're up for a sporadic fast? While spacing out meals & snacks seems to be an easy task, you can easily ruin your quick if you make these mistakes.

Intermittent fasting is a regimen that alternates between fasting and feeding periods. In contrast to most dietary philosophies, intermittent fasting focuses on when to eat rather than what to eat. Most people who follow this diet aim to consume fewer calories to lose weight.

Intermittent fasting is a lifestyle that alternates between periods of fasting (either no food or a substantial decrease in calories) and periods of uncontrolled feeding. It is encouraged to increase indicators of wellbeing that are linked to diabetes, like blood pressure & cholesterol levels, as well as to alter body structure by losing fat mass and weight. Traditional fasting, as defined in early texts by Plato, Socrates, & religious communities, is a common practice used for spiritual or health gain. 1st Fasting usually involves abstaining from food and drink for a period varying from 12 hrs. to 1 month. It could necessitate full abstinence or only enable a limited quantity of food & drink.

Intermittent fasting might not be suitable for everyone's everyday routine, especially for those who work unusually long hours or have highly active lifestyles that necessitate eating more frequently. Furthermore, there is scant and contradictory evidence that stringent dieting (of any kind) contributes to long-term, effective weight loss. Furthermore, following a rigid diet (such as extended fasting) will raise the likelihood of having an eating disorder.

This is the reason we have covered every single detail about fasting in this book which will be helpful for everyone especially women over the age of 50 years. You will get to know all the dos and don'ts in detail once you go through this book. So wait for no further and start right away to enter the enhanced world of intermittent fasting.

You will find all the necessary details, the minor's one too, once you explore this book further. For your easiness and better understanding, the book is easy to read and grasp. We have got you cover especially if you are a woman over the age of 50 but rest assured even if you are not over 50 or even if you are not even a woman still you will be able to find loads and loads of information regarding intermittent fasting and all the queries running through your mind.

Chapter 1: Intermittent Fasting and it's Working

Let us begin with this book by making you understand that what really is intermittent fasting, how does it work, and why so many people follow it? This chapter will guide you through the basics.

1.1

Intermittent Fasting

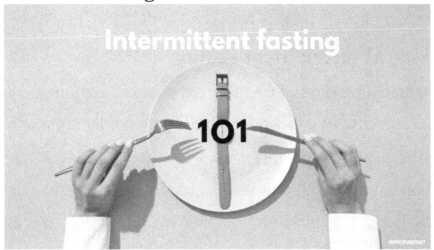

Intermittent fasting has quickly gained popularity as a food movement to watch. Intermittent fasting has been one of the most regularly quoted diets over the last two years, according to the IFIC Foundation's Food & Health Survey. What exactly is intermittent fasting, though? The diet's increasing success justifies deep dives into the basic conditions, research, and possible contemplation for attempting it.

Intermittent fasting limits whether and how frequently you consume — or both — for some time. There are many options.

Any second day, you feed regularly during alternate-day fasting. On the days in b/w, you consume just 25% of the regular calorie requirements in one meal. So, if you consumed 1,800 Cal on Monday, Wednesday, & Friday, on Tuesday, Thursday, & Saturday, you'd eat a 450-calorie lunch (and little else).

In the 5:2 diet, you feed regularly for five days and only consume just 400 500 calories for the next two days.

1.2

Every day is the same for the 16:8 method: you fast for 16 hours and only eat regularly for eight hours, such as between 9 a.m. & 5 p.m.

Working of Intermittent Fasting

Fasting on alternating days, for entire days with a certain frequency each week, or for a specific time period are the most popular approaches.

• Alternate-day fasting—alternating b/w days that you don't eat and dayswhen you eat one meal that meets around 25% of your regular calorie requirements. Fasting is observed on Mondays, Wednesdays, and Fridays, although no dietary limits are observed on alternating days.

• Whole-day fasting—1 to 2 days a week of full fasting or up to 25 percent of regular calorie requirements, with no restrictions on diet on the other days. The 5:2 diet, for example, recommends no dietary restriction five days a week, followed by a 400 to 500 calorie diet the other 2 days.

• Time-restricted eating entails sticking to a daily food schedule and fastingfor a set amount of time. Example: Meals are consumed from 8 a.m. to 3 p.m., with the rest of the day spent fasting.

What is intermittent fasting & why does it have such a large following?

Intermittent fasting is a regimen that alternates between fasting and feeding periods. In contrast to most dietary philosophies, intermittent fasting focuses on when to eat rather than what to eat. Most people who follow this diet aim to consume fewer calories to lose weight.

There is a few exceptions of this diet's feeding and fasting cycles, including a regular 16:8 ratio of fasting hours to eating hours; the 5:2 approach (5 days of eating normally & 2 days of eating 500 to 600 calories a day); & the "Eat-

1.3

Stop-Eat" method (5 days of eating normally & two days of eating 500 to 600 calories per day) (which demand fasting for 24 hours 1 to 2 times per week). Food is not permitted at this period, regardless of the duration of the fasting stage; however, coffee, tea, & water are permitted.

Intermittent fasting is a lifestyle that alternates between periods of fasting (either no food or a substantial decrease in calories) and periods of uncontrolled feeding. It is encouraged to increase indicators of wellbeing that are linked to diabetes, like blood pressure & cholesterol levels, as well as to alter body structure by losing fat mass and weight. Traditional fasting, as defined in early texts by Plato, Socrates, & religious communities, is a common practice used for spiritual or health gain. 1st Fasting usually involves abstaining from food and drink for a period varying from 12 hrs. to 1 month. It could necessitate full abstinence or only enable a limited quantity of food & drink.

Physiological changes resulting from prolonged very low Cal diets can allow the body to respond to the calorie restriction, preventing more weight loss. Intermittent fasting tries to solve this issue by cycling between lowcalorie diets for a short period accompanied by regular feeding, which can eliminate these adaptations. In terms of weight reduction performance, though, the evidence does not reliably prove the intermittent fasting is equivalent to continuous low-calorie diets.

1.4 What has been discovered by studies on intermittent fasting?

One of the most common reasons people begin a fresh diet is to lose weight, & some experts say intermittent fasting can help. In 2018, a systematic study and meta-analysis looked at whether various types of intermittent fasting would help people lose weight. Six trials were included in the study, with durations varying from three to twelve months. Four of the researchers used sustained energy limitation as a comparator mediation, which meant that subjects consumed fewer calories during the day than they would otherwise. Two of the trials featured a no-treatment placebo group, who did not make any changes to their dietary patterns. In particular, 400 overweight & obese people were studied to see if intermittent fasting affected their weight. Intermittent energy limitation was shown to be more beneficial than no therapy for weight reduction by the researchers. In terms of weight reduction, there was little distinction between periodic and constant energy restrictions. These findings are focused on a limited number of trials, and further research is required to validate the weight-loss benefits of intermittent fasting.

More recent research looked at the effects of alternate-day fasting (eating as much as you like any single day and none on the days in b/w) on calorie consumption in 60 safe and overweight people. After 4 weeks, researchers discovered that participants who fasted on alternating days consumed 37% fewer calories than they had recorded consuming before the analysis and dropped almost 8 pounds on average. The research's control group even consumed fewer calories and shed weight by adopting an "ad-lib diet" during the study. As a consequence, they consumed 8% fewer calories than they had previously recorded, and they lost almost a 1/2-lb of body mass on average. Although these findings are positive, fasting still comes with some valuable guidance. "Even stable adults do not practice alternate-day fasting after consulting a clinician to rule out harmful consequences related to serious medical conditions," the researchers concluded. A wholesome and nutritious diet is likely important to promote the positive results produced by alternate-day fasting, although this was not explicitly tested in this study."

1.5
Metabolic Health

In addition to weight loss, physical health has been mentioned as a possible advantage of intermittent fasting. Various forms of intermittent fasting regimens, as well as their possible health benefits and related physiological processes, were discussed in this study. Changes in weight and metabolic factors (e.g., blood glucose levels and overall cholesterol) correlated with type two diabetes, cardiovascular disease, & cancer were the health effects of concern. The study covered 16 human trials, the bulk of which recruited less than 50 subjects for brief periods, implying that the findings could be viewed with caution. Intermittent fasting, according to the writers of this study, can be a successful way to increase metabolic health for individuals who can comfortably go without food for long periods. "A relevant clinical and research challenge is whether following a normal, intermittent fasting program is a viable & sustainable population-based approach for improving metabolic health," they write at the end.

Composition of the body

Our body structure (the ratio of lean mass to fat mass) has health effects. Excess fat mass, for example, is harmful to one's fitness, while lean mass, such as skeletal muscle, is beneficial. This study looked at research on

1.6

intermittent fasting systems to see how successful they are at optimizing body structure and disease biomarkers. It looked at three different forms of fasting: alterative fasting, whole-day fasting, and time-restricted diet. In overweight, normal-weight, and obese individuals, alternate-day fasting studies lasting three to 12 weeks tend to be successful in lowering body fat, body weight, overall cholesterol, and triglycerides. Fasting for the whole day for 12 to 24 weeks decreased bodyweight which fat, and increased blood lipids (total triglycerides & cholesterol). Relevantly, research on time-limited feeding was found to be minimal, making it impossible to draw firm conclusions. The length and scope of these experiments are constrained. Intermittent fasting ought to be studied over longer periods to see whether it will change body structure and biomarkers linked to health.

Is there something more to think about?

Intermittent fasting might not be suitable for everyone's everyday routine, especially for those who work unusually long hours or have highly active lifestyles that necessitate eating more frequently. Furthermore, there is scant and contradictory evidence that stringent dieting (of any kind) contributes to long-term, effective weight loss. Furthermore, following a rigid diet (such as extended fasting) will raise the likelihood of having an eating disorder.

1.7
Intermittent Fasting and Women

If you're a female with fluctuating hormones or elevated levels of subjective tension (all that counts is how much anxiety you feel) IF may be another stressor that raises cortisol levels or causes them to collapse much further if you have adrenal fatigue. That is, you've been feeling a lot of pressure for a long time and haven't been able to even things out with coping strategies due to poor diet or other lifestyle patterns. Your body would eventually run out of cortisol to produce. To control existence, we need it at appropriate stages.

When you purposefully introduce a stressor for some excuse, the trick is to momentarily delete it anywhere else. That isn't always the case when anyone chooses IF. How can you juggle job & home life stressors when maintaining a high-intensity workout routine? That's a very one-sided and unbalanced scale.

Take, for example, our Olympic athletes. The majority of them practice as a career. They remain in Rio's athlete's quarters and eat meals made for athletes. They are completely focused on the minutes, if not seconds, that they can do. They teach their brains to stop multitasking to reduce tension. Their strongest performances are the product of their greatest concentration. It's the same for your body. When food and workout stressors are added to already existing stressors, the outcome can be the polar opposite of what you want.

Is it suitable for you?

Consider occasions that you go without food for extended periods. Ask yourself the following questions if you're experimenting with intermittent fasting (whether knowingly or because your dieting attitude has infiltrated into your food control):

- Do you sound like you're getting weaker or having less stamina?
- Have you noticed that the same exercises are becoming more difficult?
- Is the consistency of your sleep deteriorating?
- Do you have any trouble concentrating or focusing?
- Can you see yourself being increasingly stressed, frustrated, or forgetful?
- Is hunger causing you to be distracted?

If you answered yes to all of these questions IF is not for you at this time.

1.9
The bottom line

Despite its success, there aren't enough long-term trials to prove intermittent fasting's health benefits. For others, a time-restricted eating pattern may work, but for some, it may lead to an unhealthy relationship to food. Furthermore, since this diet does not promote or exclude particular foods or nutrients, the healthiness of an intermittent faster's diet can differ greatly. Eating types such as the Mediterranean, Nordic, MIND, and DASH diets, which have a broad range of nutritious foods and do not necessitate stringent control or elimination of those foods, are more likely to be helpful to wellbeing and simpler to maintain over time.

Chapter 2: Intermittent or Irregular Fasting for Weight Loss

Intermittent fasting, at the most basic level, essentially helps the body to utilize its surplus resources by consuming excess body fat.

It's crucial to remember that this is natural, and humans have adapted to be able to fast for shorter periods (hrs. or days) without experiencing negative health effects.

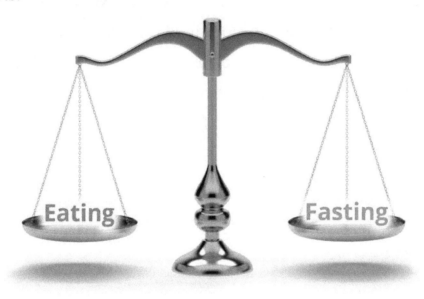

Food energy has been accumulated in the form of body fat. Your body would actually "kill" one's fat for energy if you don't eat.

Life is just about finding the right mix. The yin & the yang, the positive and the evil. The same is so when it comes to food & fasting. Overall, fasting is just the opposite of feeding. You are fasting and if you're not fed.

2.1 Here is how it works!

When we feed, we use more nutritional calories than we would use right now. Any of this electricity would have to be saved for later. Insulin is a hormone that helps the body store energy from food.

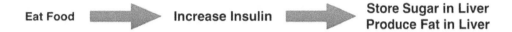

When we feed, our insulin levels increase, assisting us in storing extra energy in two respects. Carbohydrates are digested into glucose {sugar} units that can be joined together to form glycogen, which is retained in the liver or body.

However, there is a finite amount of storage capacity for sugars, and until the cap is hit, the liver begins to convert the extra glucose to fat. De-novo lipogenesis (literally "making fresh fat") is the name given to this method.

The liver stores some of the freshly produced fat, although the majority of it is distributed to other fat deposits throughout the body. While this is a more difficult procedure, the amount of fat that can be generated is almost limitless.

In our muscles, we have 2 complimentary diet energy storage mechanisms. One is simple to access but has minimal storage space (glycogen), while the other is more complex to access but has almost infinite storage space (glucose) (body fat).

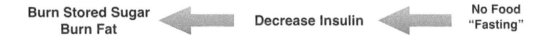

When we don't chew, the mechanism reverses. Insulin levels drop, signaling the body to begin burning accumulated energy because food is no longer accessible. Since blood glucose levels are dropping, the body must now draw glucose from storage to burn energy.

Glycogen has been the most readily available form of electricity. To supply sugar to the bodies of other cells, it is decomposed into glucose molecules. This will last for 24 to 36 hrs. and have enough energy to meet much of the body's needs. After that, the body's primary source of nutrition would be the fat breakdown.

So there are only two conditions in which the body may exist: fed and fasted. We are either storing food resources (increasing stores) or consuming stored energy (burning stored energy) (decreasing stores). It's either this or that. There can be no net weight difference if feeding & fasting are matched.

We waste nearly half of our life in the fed condition whether we start feeding as soon as we get out of bed & don't pause before we go to sleep. We may accumulate weight over time because we haven't given our bodies enough energy to destroy stored food fat.

We will just need to maximize the period we spend burning food energy to regain balance or lose weight.

Intermittent fasting, in turn, enables the body to utilize the remaining fat. What's essential to remember is there's nothing wrong with it. That is the way our bodies are made. Horses, seals, & tigers all do this. That's what people do.

Your body can constantly utilize the arriving food resources if you feed every 3rd hrs. Which is frequently advised. It might not be enough to burn much if any, body fat. You may be simply storing fat.

The body may be storing it until a moment when you won't be able to feed.

If this occurs, you are out of control. You're missing out on intermittent fasting.

Chapter 3: For Women Over 50, the Advantages of Intermittent Fasting

Intermittent fasting seems to have a wide range of health effects. The flip of a metabolic switch may potentially cause these results.

"Fasting causes glucose {blood sugar} levels to drop. Since converting fat into ketones, the body utilizes fat rather than glucose as a source of energy "Kathy McManus, head of the Dept. of Nutrition at the Harvard-affiliated Brigham & Women's Hospital, says. The switch of ketones from glucose as an energy source has a positive impact on body chemistry.

Animals who fast regularly lose weight, have lower blood pressure & heart rates, have fewer insulin resistance, have lower "poor" LDL cholesterol levels, & higher "healthy" HDL cholesterol levels, & have less inflammation. Improved memory has also been discovered in several trials.

At least in mammals, intermittent fasting is linked to a longer lifespan.

What is the reason for this? Intermittent fasting, according to a recent Harvard study, can enable each cell's energy-producing engine (mitochondria) to generate energy efficiently & maintain a more youthful state.

"When feeding throughout the day, you are not pushing the mitochondria at night, because they're meant to be doing other stuff," says Dr. William Mair, a Harvard TH. Chan School of Public researcher & assistant professor of genetics & complex diseases. "However, we also have a lot of unanswered questions."

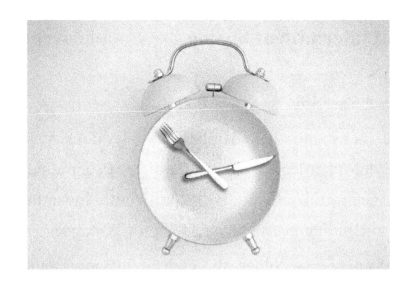

3.1 Benefits of intermittent fasting for women over 50

- Prime Females
- Tuesday, September 3rd

Lower appetite, achy muscles, decreased body density, & even sleep problems all render it harder to lose weight after 50. Simultaneously, losing weight, including harmful belly fat, will significantly lower the risk of major health problems including heart attacks, diabetes, & cancer.

Of necessity, when you get older, the chances of contracting a variety of diseases rise. When it comes to weight reduction and that the risk of contracting age-related ailments, intermittent fasting of women over 50 can be a physical fountain of youth in certain situations.

3.2 What is the process of intermittent fasting?

You won't have to deprive yourself if you practice intermittent fasting, also known as IF. It also doesn't owe you permission to eat a bunch of fatty food while you aren't fasting. Instead of consuming meals & treats during the day, you feed over a set time.

The majority of citizens adhere to an IF regimen that allows them to fast for twelve to sixteen hours a day. They enjoy regular meals & treats the majority of the day. Since often people sleep for around eight hours during their fasting hours, sticking to this feeding window isn't as difficult as it seems. You're often allowed to consume zero-calorie beverages like wine, tea, & coffee.

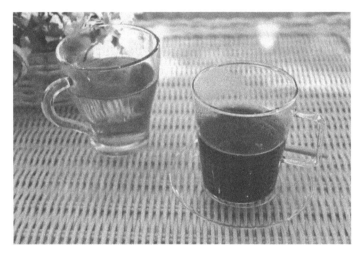

For the strongest intermittent fasting outcomes, build an eating routine that fits you. Include the following example:

- **12-hour fasts:** A 12-hour sprint entails skipping breakfast & waiting for lunch to feed. You might eat an earlier supper & skip evening snacks if you want to eat your early breakfast. A 12-12 quick is relatively simple to maintain for older women.

- **16-hour fasts:** A 16 to 8 IF schedule will help you achieve faster performance. Within an 8-hrs. span, most people prefer to eat two meals & a snack or two. For e.g., the eating window may be fixed between noon & 8 p.m., or between 8 a.m. and 4 p.m.

- **5-2 routine:** You might not be able to stick to a restricted eating schedule every day. Another choice is to follow a 12 or 16-hour quick for five days & then rest for two days. For example, you might do intermittent fasting throughout the week & eat regularly on the weekends.

- **Alternate-day fasts:** Another choice is to eat very little cal on alternate days. For instance, you might restrict your calories to under 500 calories one day & then eat normally next one. It's worth noting that regular IF fasts never necessitate calorie restrictions that low.

- You'll have the strongest effects from this diet if you stick to it. Around the same period, on rare days, you should certainly take a break from this type of eating routine. You should try different types of intermittent fasting to see which one is well for you. Many people begin their IF journey with the 12 to 12 plan and then move to the 16 to 8 plan. After that, continue to adhere to the schedule as closely as possible.

3.3
What causes intermittent fasting to be effective?

Some people claim that IF has helped them lose weight mainly because the short eating window forces them to eat fewer calories. For example, instead of three meals and two snacks, they can only have time for two meals & one snack. They become more conscious of the foods they eat and prefer to avoid fatty fats, artificial carbohydrates, & empty calories.

Of course, you have the freedom to choose any nutritious foods you choose. While certain people use intermittent fasting to limit their daily calorie consumption, some use it in conjunction with a vegan, keto, or other diets.

When you're fasting intermittently, these are the foods you can eat.

3.4

Women's intermittent fasting benefits may go beyond calorie restrictions

Although some nutritionists believe that IF only succeeds that it encourages people to eat less, others argue. They assume that with the same number of calories & other nutrients, intermittent fasting produces greater effects than traditional meal plans. Studies have also proposed that fasting for many hours a day accomplishes more than mere calorie restriction.

These are some of the metabolic modifications that IF induces, which can further explain the synergistic effects:

- **Insulin:** Lower insulin levels during the fasting cycle will aid fat burning.
- **Human Growth Hormone (HGH):** As insulin levels fall, HGH levels increase, promoting fat burning & muscle growth.
- **Noradrenaline:** When your stomach is empty, your nervous system sends this chemical to your cells to tell them you need to conserve fat for food.

Is intermittent fasting beneficial to your health?

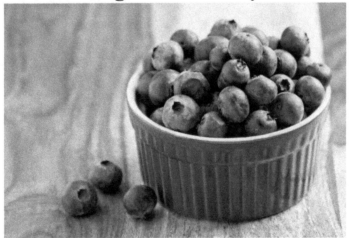

Is overnight fasting a healthy way to eat? Remember that you can just fast for 12 to 16 hours at a time, not for days. You also have plenty of time to eat a delicious and nutritious meal. Of course, certain older ladies may need

3.5

regular eating due to metabolic diseases or drug guidelines. Under any scenario, you can talk to the doctor about your dietary patterns before making any adjustments.

Although it isn't fasting, some physicians claim that allowing easy-to-digest foods like whole fruit mostly during the fasting window has health benefits. Modifications like this will also provide a much-needed break for the digestive and metabolic systems. For example, the famous weight-loss book "Fit for Life" recommended consuming just fruit after supper & before lunch.

In reality, according to the writers of this novel, they have patients who just modified their eating patterns by fasting for 12 to 16 hours per day. Despite not adhering to the diet's other guidelines or counting calories, they shed weight & improved their fitness. This technique may have failed largely because dieters swapped fast food for whole foods. In either scenario, participants considered this dietary modification to be beneficial and simple to implement. Traditionalists won't name this fasting, so it's good to remember that you have choices if you can't go without eating for more than a few hours.

3.6 Intermittent fasting typical results

In the medical literature, Dr. Becky, a chiropractor & over-50 wellness coach, claims it's difficult to identify any drawbacks to IF. She demonstrated that the blood sugar & insulin levels would drop to dangerously low levels throughout the fasting cycle. Your body will depend on stored fat for energy if insulin's hormonal fat-storing signal is not present.

The National Library of Medicine has also released an analysis of women's health-related sporadic quick outcomes. Studies on the usage of fasting as a method to minimize the incidence of cancer, diabetes, & other metabolic disorders, as well as cardiac failure, are among the report's highlights.

3.7 Is intermittent fasting (if) the best fat-loss tool?

In either scenario, IF seems to succeed mostly because it is relatively simple to follow. By reducing eating windows, they say it makes them automatically reduce calories and make healthier food decisions. According to some research, IF tends to encourage fat loss while sparing muscle mass, making it a safer option than just reducing carbs, calories, or fat.

Of note, the majority of people combine IF with some weight-loss strategy. To lose weight, you might plan to consume 1,200 calories a day. It could be cheaper to spread out 1,200 cal over two meals and two snacks rather than three meals and three snacks. If you've had trouble losing weight because your diet didn't fit or was too difficult to adhere to, you may want to consider intermittent fasting.

Dr. Kathryn Waldrep advocates feeding during an eight-hour timeframe and selecting the period depending on the body's circadian cycles in Prime Women's newly introduced PLATE weight loss program. Eat b/w 9 a.m. & 5 p.m. whether you're an early riser. Night owls will consume their first meal around midday and their last meal around 8:00 p.m. There seems to be credible data about the validity of this method to eating for weight loss as further studies on whether and circadian cycles are conducted.

Sue Ryskamp, a dietitian at the University of Michigan, discusses the effects of intermittent fasting, who it is ideal for, & how to get started.

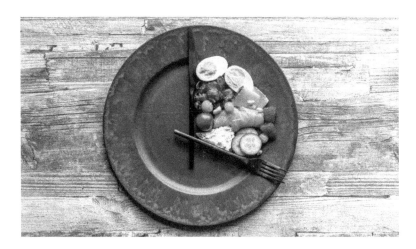

Weight loss is daunting, or could intermittent fasting aid in the process? This eating style, which includes fasting and eating loops, is gaining popularity as the study shows that when it comes to losing weight, it's not only what you consume, but what you eat.

Individuals utilize specific times of eating — usually within an eight-to-10hour timeframe — to shed weight during intermittent fasting, according to Michigan Medicine dietitian, who sees patients at the Frankel Cardiovascular Center at U-M.

"So if our insulin levels go down high enough & for long enough as they do during a fasting cycle, we can burn off fat," she notes.

When an individual does not eat, their insulin levels decrease. Reduced insulin levels allow cells to release accumulated glucose as energy during a fasting cycle. Weight reduction is achieved by repeating this procedure daily, similar to extended fasting. "Besides, this form of fasting also leads to a lower average calorie intake, which aids in weight loss," Ryskamp adds.

When fasting, intermittent fasting helps the GI tract to relax and rebuild itself. "This is because the body can utilize fat contained in your cells as food, causing you to eat fat rather than retain it, resulting in weight loss,"

Ryskamp explains. "Recent research findings are encouraging, especially when paired with exercise & a plant-based diet like the Mediterranean diet."

Chapter 4: Frequently Asked Questions About Intermittent Fasting

Following are some queries that one may wonder while going through intermittent fasting.

4.1 What is the mechanism behind intermittent fasting?

The plan fits better if you quit feeding at a specific time of day and don't feed at all at night. That implies no snacks in between or before bed. While feeding times vary from individual to individual, all patients have improved eating between the hours of 10 a.m. and 6 p.m.

4.2

Is it a challenging diet to follow?

Intermittent fasting may be challenging at first, however, when the body transitions to a different way of eating, the diet becomes more manageable. The end goal is to become more conscious of what & where you consume. It establishes guidelines and standards, which many patients appreciate.

We recommend regular fitness, eliminating calories, and eating fruits, herbs, beans, whole grains, lentils, lean proteins, and good fats in addition to intermittent fasting.

4.4

4.3 When is the most appropriate moment to fast?

Fat burning usually starts after 12 hours of fasting & increases between 16 & 24 hours of fasting.

Is this fasting prescribed for how many days a week?

People usually swift for up to 16 hrs. a day. This is normally accomplished by missing breakfast the next morning after consuming the prior day's last dinner. Intermittent fasting is a pattern that entails going without eating for 24 hours up to two days per week.

4.6
What is the maximum amount of food I can consume during the feeding period?

If you choose to lose weight, stick to a calorie intake that allows you to lose 1-2 pounds every week. You'll need to eat off 500 calories a day on average to drop one pound per week.

4.7

Is there some kind of beverage that should drink during the fast?

It's more in the water... and there's a lot of it. If you're going to fast, make sure you drink plenty of water during the time you're not consuming solid food. Broth made from vegetables, chicken, or bones may also be eaten. Caffeine-containing drinks, such as soda, can be stopped.

4.8

Are there any other advantages of intermittent fasting besides weight loss?

Fasting can lower cholesterol, increase carbohydrate regulation, minimize liver fat, and raise blood pressure, in addition to lowering body weight. Patients report greater stamina, enhanced muscle control, and more sleep. Eating under the circadian cycle (eat during the day, sleep at night) aids in the promotion of sleep state. Fasting, which results in dietary restriction, has also been found to extend the lifetime of even healthier people in studies. Fasting has also been linked to a reduction in tumor development and the prevention of breast cancer recurrence, according to research.

4.9

Can it entail calorie counting?

Not actually, but if you skip treats before bedtime and go longer hours without feeding, the calorie intake can decrease. You're still eating things that are usually lower in calories while you eat a predominantly plant-based diet.

4.10
Who is the most benefited from intermittent fasting?

Irregular fasting isn't suitable for anyone. This is another item to include in the toolkit for those who have tried to lose weight. In the end, it comes down to a person's lifestyle & the decisions he or she makes. They must consider their choices and determine, "What would be best for me?"

4.11

Is there any need to stop intermittent fasting if you have a medical condition?

People with brittle diabetes, people with a background of eating problems such as anorexia & bulimia, & breastfeeding or pregnant women do not fast unless they are closely monitored by a specialist.

4.12
Intermittent fasting explained in human terms

Intermittent fasting is one of the most common health and wellness phenomena on the planet.

It entails fasting & feeding loops that alternate.

Many trials have shown that this will help you lose weight, increase your cardiovascular fitness, shield you from cancer, and maybe even help you live longer.

This section outlines what intermittent fasting is and why it's essential to pay attention to it.

4.13
De-Intermittent Fasting?

Intermittent fasting is an eating practice under which you alternate between eating and fasting times.

It does not specify the foods should be consumed, but rather when they should be consumed.

There are a variety of intermittent fasting strategies available, many of which divide the day or week into feeding and fasting times.

The majority of people still "fast" while sleeping every day. Extending the fast can be an easy way to practice intermittent fasting.

Miss breakfast, eat the first lunch at midday, and the last meal at 8:00 pm to do this.

Then you're fasting for 16 hrs. a day, with an 8-hour feeding time. The 16/8 approach is the most widely used type of intermittent fasting.

Intermittent fasting is very easy, contrary to popular belief. During a fast, several people feel healthier and getting more energy.

Hunger is normally not a challenge, but it may be at the beginning when the body adjusts to not feeding for long periods.

During the fasting time, no food is permitted, although water, coffee, tea, & other non-caloric drinks are permitted.

During the fasting time, certain types of intermittent fasting provide for limited quantities of low-calorie foods.

Taking vitamins when fasting is normally permitted as long as they provide no calories.

4.14

Intermittent fasting (or "IF") is an eating practice in which you alternate between eating and fasting times. It's a common health & wellness theme that's backed up by science.

Tools for healthcare

Choose a diet that is perfect for you.

Based on your responses to three fast questions, our free evaluation lists the right diets for you.

Why Fast?

Fasting has been practiced by humans for 1000 years. When there was absolutely no food left, it was sometimes done out of desperation.

It was often undertaken for religious purposes in some cases. Fasting is required by many faiths, including Islam, Christianity, and Buddhism.

When humans & other animals are ill, they always respond quickly.

Fasting is not "unnatural," because our bodies are well capable of going without food for long periods.

When we don't feed for a while, our bodies go through a variety of changes to help us to survive during a drought. Hormones, chromosomes, and critical cellular repair pathways are all involved.

When we fast, our blood sugar and insulin levels drop significantly, whilst our levels of human growth hormone skyrocket.

Many people use intermittent fasting to reduce weight and it is a quick and easy way to cut calories & burn fat.

Others use so to increase their physiological health and may improve a variety of risk factors & health indicators.

4.15

Intermittent fasting has also been seen to help people live longer. It may prolong the lifespan as effective as calorie restriction in rodents, according to studies.

It can also help guard against diseases such as heart failure, type 2 diabetes, stroke, Alzheimer's disease, among others, according to some studies.

Others like extended fasting because it is more convenient.

It's a useful "life hack" that helps you simplify your life while still optimizing your fitness. Your life would be easier if you just have to prepare a few meals.

It also saves time not needing to feed 3-4 times a day (with all the cooking and cleaning it entails). There was a variety of it.

Chapter 5: Types of Intermittent Fasting

In recent years, intermittent fasting seems to be quite common, and many various types/methods have arisen. Here are a few of the most well-known:

- **The 16/8 Method:** Feed only between noon & 8:00 p.m. for 16 hours per day.
- **Eat-Stop-Eat:** Do not eat something from dinner 1 day to dinner the next day once or twice a week (a 24 hour fast).
- **The 5:2 Diet:** Consume just 500 to 600 calories on 2 days of a week.

And there is a slew of other options.

Intermittent fasting can be done in a variety of ways. The 16/8 process, EatStop-Eat, & the 5:2 diet are the most common.

Take-Home Message

Restricting the feeding window & fasting on occasion may have some really impressive health effects as long as you adhere to nutritious foods.

It's an efficient way to reduce weight and boost metabolic fitness while still simplifying your life.

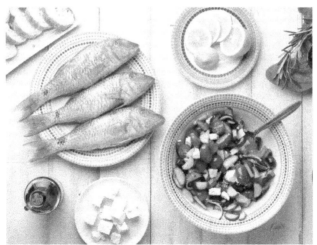

How Intermittent Fasting Can Help You Lose Weight?

- Fasting Plans
- Hormonal Impact
- Weight Loss
- Muscle Preservation
- Healthier Eating
- Tips
- Conclusion

There are several approaches to losing weight.

Intermittent fasting is a technique that has gained popularity in recent years.

Daily, short-term fasts — or times of little or no food intake — are part of an eating trend known as intermittent fasting.

Intermittent fasting is commonly thought of as a weight-loss strategy. People that fast for brief amounts of time consumes fewer calories, which can take to weight loss with time.

Intermittent fasting, on the other hand, can help reduce risk factors for diabetes and cardiovascular disease by reducing blood sugar & cholesterol.

All that you need to understand about intermittent fasting & weight reduction is covered in this chapter.

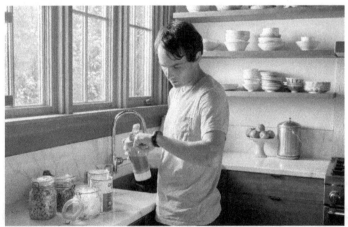

5.1 What effect does intermittent fasting have on the hormones?

While intermittent fasting can help one's lose weight, it can also have a negative impact on your hormones.

This is due to the fact that body fat is just the body's means of retaining resources (calories).

When you don't feed, the body goes through a series of adjustments in order to allow the accumulated resources more available.

Variations in nervous system function, as well as significant changes in the rates of many important hormones, are examples. When you quick, the metabolism shifts in two ways:

- **Insulin** is a hormone that regulates blood sugar levels. While you feed, your insulin levels rise, & when you fast, your insulin levels plummet. Insulin levels that are lower aid fat burning.

- **Norepinephrine (norepinephrine).** Norepinephrine is a neurotransmitter that causes fat cells to dissolve body fat to free fatty acid which can be burnt for energy.

Interestingly, short-term fasting can increase fat burning, contrary to what some advocates of eating 5–6 meals a day say.

Alternate-day fasting tests of 3 to12 weeks, and also whole-day fasting tests of 12–24 weeks, have been shown to lower body weight & body fat.

Still, further study into the long-term consequences of intermittent fasting is required.

Human growth hormone (HGH) is another hormone that changes during a high, with levels rising to five-fold.

HGH was formerly thought to aid fat burning, but recent evidence suggests it may warn the brain to save resources, rendering weight loss more difficult.

HGH can increase appetite and decrease energy metabolism by stimulating a limited population of agouti-related protein neurons.

Fasting for a short period of time causes a number of physiological modifications that aid weight loss. Nonetheless, rising HGH levels can have an indirect effect on energy metabolism, making it difficult to maintain weight loss.

5.2 Intermittent fasting aids in calorie reduction and weight loss

Intermittent fasting lets you consume fewer calories, which is why it helps you lose weight.

During the fasting times, many of the procedures include missing meals.

You can consume fewer calories unless you remunerate by having even more during eating hours.

Intermittent fasting decreased body weight by 3 to 8% during a span of 3– 24 weeks, according to a 2014 study.

Intermittent fasting can result in a weight loss of 0.55 to 1.65 lbs. (0.25 to 0.75 kg) per week, depending on the degree of weight loss.

The waist circumference of the participants decreased by 4–7%, meaning that they reduced belly fat.

These findings suggest how intermittent fasting may be an effective weightloss strategy.

However, the advantages of intermittent fasting extend well beyond weight reduction.

It also has many metabolic health effects and can also reduce the likelihood of cardiovascular disease.

While calorie counting is not necessary when having intermittent fasting, losing weight is mostly induced by a decrease in total calorie intake.

When calories are balanced between classes, studies contrasting intermittent fasting & constant calorie restriction find little difference in weight loss.

Intermittent fasting is a simple way to shed pounds without having to count calories. Many trials have shown that it can aid in weight loss and the reduction of belly fat.

5.3

When dieting, intermittent fasting can help you preserve muscle mass

Dieting has the unfortunate side effect of causing muscle loss as well as fat loss.

Intermittent fasting has been found in several research to be effective for retaining muscle mass when losing body fat.

Intermittent calorie limitations resulted in comparable weight loss as constant calorie restriction, albeit with a far lower loss in muscle mass, according to a clinical study.

Just 10% of the weight loss in the periodic calorie restriction trials was muscle mass, while 25% of the weight loss in the calorie restriction studies was muscle mass.

Take the results with a grain of salt, though, that these experiments have certain shortcomings. When opposed to other forms of diet schedules, more modern findings have shown little changes in muscle mass or lean mass for intermittent fasting.

Although some research shows that intermittent fasting, as opposed to traditional calorie restriction, may help you keep further muscle mass, more recent findings have refuted this theory.

Good food is easier with intermittent fasting

One of the primary advantages of intermittent fasting is its ease, according to many people.

Many intermittent fasting diets only enable you to keep track of time rather than calories.

5.4

The right eating plan for you is one that you will maintain with time. Intermittent fasting would have clear advantages for long-term wellness and weight loss as it allows it easier for one's to adhere to a balanced diet.

Intermittent fasting has a number of advantages, including making healthier eating easier. In the long term, this can make maintaining a balanced diet simpler.

5.5
How to Succeed With an Intermittent Fasting Protocol

If you intend to lose weight through intermittent fasting, there are a few points to bear in mind:

1. **The consistency of the food.** It's always essential to consume healthy foods. Eat single-ingredient, whole foods as much as possible.

2. **Calories** are also relevant. During non-fasting hours, choose to consume normally, just not so often that you substitute for the calories you lost when fasting.

3. **Durability.** If you want it to succeed, you must stay with it for a long time, much like every other weight losing tool.

4. **Patience** may take some time for the body to respond to an intermittent fasting regimen. It would get better if you are consistent to your meal plan.

Exercise, such as weight exercise, is recommended in virtually all common intermittent fasting protocols. If you choose to burn mostly body fat while retaining your muscle mass, this is key.

When it comes to intermittent fasting, calorie counting is normally not important at first. Calorie counting, on the other hand, maybe helpful if the weight reduction plateaus.

If you choose to lose weight with extended fasting, you must always eat well and sustain a calorie deficit. Consistency is important, as is regular exercise.

Finally, extended fasting may be an effective weight-loss strategy.

Its weight loss is largely due to a decrease in calorie consumption, although some of its hormone-related benefits which also play a role.

5.6

Intermittent fasting isn't for everybody, however, it may be incredibly helpful for others.

Common intermittent fasting techniques

Intermittent fasting has been a common health practice in recent years. It's said to help people lose weight, boost their metabolic fitness, and maybe even live longer.

This eating trend may be approached in a variety of ways.

Any strategy has the potential to be successful, but deciding which one works better for you is a personal decision.

Intermittent fasting can be achieved in six separate forms.

5.7

Selecting an intermittent fasting program

Intermittent fasting can be done in a variety of ways. Among the most common are:

- The 16:8 framework
- The 5:2 eating plan
- Warrior's Diet
- Eat Stop Eat
- Fasting on alternating days (ADF)
- Unplanned Meal skipping

All strategies may be useful, but determining which one works better for you is a personal decision.

Here's a rundown of the benefits and drawbacks of each approach to help you decide which is best for you.

1. The16/8 method

One of the most common fasting plans for weight loss was its 16/8 intermittent fasting method.

Food & calorie-containing drinks are limited to 8 hours a day under the package. It necessitates fasting for the remaining 16 hrs. of the day.

While other diets have rigid guidelines and regulations, the 16/8 approach is more versatile and is focused on such a time-restricted feeding (TRF) model.

You can consume calories every 8 hours.

Few individuals stop feeding late and keep to a 9:00 a.m. to 5:00 p.m. plan, while others miss breakfast & fast from noon to 8:00 p.m.

5.8

Limiting the amount of hours you may eat throughout the day can aid in weight loss and blood pressure reduction.

According to research, time-restricted eating habits, such as the 16/8 cycle, can help avoid hypertension and decrease food consumption, resulting in weight loss.

In a 2016 report, the 16/8 approach was shown to help reduce body mass and retain muscle mass to male subjects when paired with resistance exercise.

More recent research discovered that the 16/8 approach has little impact on muscle or power increases in women doing resistance exercises.

Although the 16/8 approach may be quickly incorporated into any lifestyle, certain people may find it difficult to go 16 hours without food.

Furthermore, consuming so many chips or unhealthy food during the 8-hour fasting time will counteract the benefits of 16/8 intermittent fasting.

To reap the most nutritional benefits from this diet, consume a wellbalanced diet rich in fruits, whole grains, vegetables, healthy fats, & protein.

THE 16/8 METHOD

	DAY 1	DAY 2	DAY 3	DAY 4	DAY 5	DAY 6	DAY 7
Midnight 4 AM 8 AM	FAST	FAST	FAST	FAST	FAST	FAST	FAST
12 PM	First meal	First meal	First meal	First meal	First meal	First meal	First meal
4 PM	Last meal by 8pm	Last meal by 8pm	Last meal by 8pm	Last meal by 8pm	Last meal by 8pm	Last meal by 8pm	Last meal by 8pm
8 PM Midnight	FAST	FAST	FAST	FAST	FAST	FAST	FAST

The 16/8 method entails fasting for 14 to 16 hours a day and limiting your feeding window to 8 to 10 hours.

You may consume 2, 3, or even 4 meals during the feeding time.

Fitness guru Martin Berkhan popularized this form, which is also recognized as Lean gains protocol.

It's as simple as not consuming something after dinner & missing breakfast to adopt this fasting process.

If you have your final meal at 8:00 pm and don't eat again before noon the day after, you'll have fasted for 16 hours.

Women are usually advised to fast for just 14 to 15 hours since they tend to perform well with shorter fasts.

This approach can be challenging to adapt to at first for those who get truly hungry & like to consume breakfast. Many breakfast-skippers, on the other side, feed in this fashion instinctively.

During the quick, you can drink coffee, water, & other low-calorie drinks to make you feel less hungry.

It's important to focus on consuming nutritious foods across your eating periods. If you eat a lot of junk food or ingest an unhealthy amount of calories, this approach would not work.

Fasting for 16 hrs. For men & 14 to15 hrs. For women on a regular basis. Every day, you'll limit the feeding to 8 to10 hrs. Span during that you should take in two meals. Three or more meals.

2. The 5:2 diet

The 5:2 diet is a simple intermittent fasting strategy.

You eat regularly five days a week and don't count calories. Then you cut your calorie consumption to 1/4 of your normal requirements for the remaining 2 days of the week.

For anyone who eats 2,000 calories a day on a daily basis, this will include cutting their calorie consumption to 500 calories two days a week.

According to a survey published in 2018,

According to a Recent Study, the 5:2 diet is almost as good for weight reduction and blood glucose management in people with type 2 diabetes as daily calorie restriction.

Another research showed also that the 5:2 diet was almost as good for weight control and the treatment of metabolic disorders including cardiac failure and diabetes as constant calorie restriction.

The 5:2 diet allows you to choose which days one's fast, & there are no restrictions to whether or what you consume of full-calorie days.

It's worth noting, though, that eating "normally" on a full-calorie day does not imply that you can consume anything you want.

And though it's just for two days a week, limiting yourself to 500 calories a day is difficult. Furthermore, eating too little calories can cause you to become faint or ill.

While the 5:2 diet may be beneficial, it is not for all. Consult a physician to see whether the 5:2 diet is right for you.

THE 5:2 DIET

DAY 1	DAY 2	DAY 3	DAY 4	DAY 5	DAY 6	DAY 7
Eats normally	Women: 500 calories Men: 600 calories	Eats normally	Eats normally	Women: 500 calories Men: 600 calories	Eats normally	Eats normally

The 5:2 diet includes eating regularly 5 days a week and limiting your calorie consumption to 500 to 600 calories on the remaining two days.

Michael Mosley, a British writer, popularized this diet, which is also regarded as the Easy Diet.

On fasting days, women should consume 500 calories & men should consume 600 calories.

You can, for example, eat regularly every day except Mondays & Thursdays. You consume 2 minor meals of 250 Cal for only women & 300 Cal each for men for those two days.

There are no trials evaluating the 5:2 diet specifically, as opponents rightly point out, but there are loads of studies about the advantages of intermittent fasting.

Diet entails consuming 500 to 600 calories two days a week and 500 to 600 calories the rest of the week. The remaining 5 days

3.   Eat Stop Eat

Brad Pilon, who wrote the book "Eat Stop Eat," popularized an unorthodox solution to intermittent fasting called "Eat Stop Eat."

This intermittent fasting schedule entails deciding on 1 or 2 nonconsecutive days a week that you can go without food for a 24-hour cycle.

You can consume as much as you like the rest of the week, so it's best to eat a well-balanced diet to stop overindulging.

A weekly 24-hrs. fast is justified by the belief that eating less calories would result in weight loss.

Fasting for up to 24 hrs. will induce a metabolic change, causing the body to use fat instead of glucose as an energy source.

However, abstaining from food for 24 hrs. at a time takes a ton of effort which may contribute to bingeing and overeating afterward. It may even result in disordered eating habits.

To ascertain the Eat Stop Eat diet's possible health benefits & weight-losing properties, further study is required.

Before you try Eat Stop Eat, talk to the doctor to see if it's a good weightloss plan for you.

Fitness specialist Brad Pilon popularized this form, which has been very popular in a few years.

This amounts to a complete 24-hour fast if you fast from dinner 1 day to dinners the next day.

You've done a perfect 24-hour quick if you end dinner at 7:00 p.m. Monday & don't feed again before dinner at 7 p.m. Tuesday. The final result is the same if you fast from lunch to lunch or breakfast to breakfast.

During the short, liquids such as coffee, water, and other low-calorie drinks are tolerated, but solid foods are not.

It's important that you diet normally during the feeding cycles while you're attempting to lose weight. In other words, one's can consume as much as you would if you weren't fasting at all.

A complete 24-hrs. Fast can be challenging for certain citizens, which is a possible disadvantage to this approach. You don't have to go all for right away, however. It's perfect, to begin with 14 to 16 hours, and work your way up.

One to two 24-hour fasts a week as part of an intermittent fasting regimen.

4.   Fasting on alternating days

Alterative fasting is a simple, easy-to-follow intermittent fasting plan. You speed every single day on this diet, so you can consume anything you desire on the non-fasting day.

On fasting days, certain variations of this diet follow an "updated" fasting approach that includes consuming about 500 calories. Some models, on the other hand, fully exclude calories on fasting days.

Fasting on alternate days has been shown to help people lose weight.

In a randomized pilot trial of adults with obesity, alternate-day fasting was shown to be as beneficial for weight reduction as everyday calorie restriction.

Another research showed that after transitioning between 36 hrs. of fasting & 12 hrs. of unlimited feeding for four weeks, participants ate 35% less calories and lost a total of 7.7 lbs. (3.5 kg).

If you're serious about losing weight, incorporating a workout routine into your daily routine will improve.

According to research, mixing alternate-day fasting to endurance training will result in weight loss that is twice as effective as strictly fasting.

Fasting for a full day any other day can be challenging, particularly if you're new to the practice. On non-fasting days, it's simple to go overboard.

If you're unfamiliar to intermittent fasting, start with a changed fasting schedule to relax into alternate-day fasting.

It's better to eat a healthy diet, including good protein foods & low-calorie veggies to make you feel whole, whether you begin with a relaxed fasting schedule or a complete quick.

ALTERNATE-DAY FASTING

DAY 1	DAY 2	DAY 3	DAY 4	DAY 5	DAY 6	DAY 7
Eats normally	24-hour fast OR Eat only a few hundred calories	Eats normally	24-hour fast OR Eat only a few hundred calories	Eats normally	24-hour fast OR Eat only a few hundred calories	Eats normally

You fast the single day as you observe alternate-day fasting.

This approach is available in a number of ways. During fasting days, some of them make around 500 calories.

This technique was used in several of the test-tube experiments that demonstrated the health effects of intermittent fasting.

A complete fast any other day may seem excessive, so it is not suggested for beginners.

This approach can cause you to go to bed hungry many days a week, which is inconvenient and unlikely to be sustainable.

Alterative fasting entails going without food or taking just a few small meals every other day hundred calories.

5.   The Warrior Diet

The Warrior Diet is really an intermittent fasting regimen inspired by ancient warriors' dietary habits.

The Warrior Diet, developed by Ori Hofmekler in 2001, is more severe than the 16:8 approach but less rigid than the Feed Quick Eat method.

It entails consuming very little throughout the day for 20 hours & then eating as frequently as needed during a 4-hour time at night.

During the 20-hour fast, the Warrior Diet allows dieters to eat limited quantities of animal ingredients, hard-boiled eggs, fresh fruits & vegetables, and also non-calorie beverages.

People can eat whatever they want for a 4-hrs window after a 20-hour short, but unprocessed, nutritious, & organic foods are preferred.

Although no study has been done on the Warrior Diet directly, human trials have shown that time-restricted eating periods can result in weight loss.

Other health benefits of time-restricted feeding periods are unknown. In mice, time-restricted feeding cycles have been shown to inhibit diabetes, slow tumor growth, postpone aging, and extend lifespan.

More analysis on a Warrior Diet is required to truly comprehend its weightloss advantages.

The Warrior Diet can be impossible to stick to since it limits calorie intake to just 4 hours a day. Overeating late at night is really a common issue.

The Warrior Diet has been linked to eating disorders. If you're up for a challenge, see a physician and see if it's correct for you.

Intermittent fasting comes with a variety of forms, each with its own set of advantages and drawbacks. Consult the doctor to determine which solution is best for you.

THE WARRIOR DIET

	DAY 1	DAY 2	DAY 3	DAY 4	DAY 5	DAY 6	DAY 7
Midnight							
4 AM	Eating only small amounts of vegetables and fruits	Eating only small amounts of vegetables and fruits	Eating only small amounts of vegetables and fruits	Eating only small amounts of vegetables and fruits	Eating only small amounts of vegetables and fruits	Eating only small amounts of vegetables and fruits	Eating only small amounts of vegetables and fruits
8 AM							
12 PM							
4 PM	Large meal	Large meal	Large meal	Large meal	Large meal	Large meal	Large meal
8 PM							
Midnight							

During the day, you consume tiny quantities of raw fruits and vegetables, and at night, you eat one big meal.

Basically, one's fast through the day and feeds within a 4-hour feeding span at night.

One of the first common diets to incorporate a type of intermittent fasting was the Warrior Diet.

The food preferences on this diet are somewhat close to those on the paleo diet, consisting entirely of the whole, unprocessed ingredients.

The Warrior Diet promotes a healthy lifestyle. During the day, consuming just tiny quantities of vegetables & fruits, then eating one big meal at night.

6.   Unplanned Meal skipping

SPONTANEOUS MEAL SKIPPING

DAY 1	DAY 2	DAY 3	DAY 4	DAY 5	DAY 6	DAY 7
Breakfast	Skipped Meal	Breakfast	Breakfast	Breakfast	Breakfast	Breakfast
Lunch	Lunch	Lunch	Lunch	Lunch	Lunch	Lunch
Dinner	Dinner	Dinner	Dinner	Skipped Meal	Dinner	Dinner

You don't have to stick to a strict intermittent fasting schedule to enjoy any of the advantages. Another choice is to miss meals on occasion, as when you aren't hungry or when you are too distracted to prepare and eat.

It's a fallacy that people must feed every few hrs. or risk malnutrition or muscle loss. Your body is designed to endure long stretches of starvation, let alone missing 1 or 2 meals every now and then.

As a consequence, if you're not hungry 1 day, miss breakfast & have a good lunch & dinner instead. Alternatively, if you're traveling and can't locate something you want to consume, go on a quick fast.

A random sporadic fast is when you skip 1 or 2 meals when one's feel like it.

During other meals, make sure you consume nutritious snacks.

Missing one or two meals is another way to exercise intermittent fasting.

If you don't feel like eating or don't have time to feed

5.8 Health line Diet Score: 3.96 out of 5

A type of eating is intermittent fasting that involves fasting on a regular basis.

The 5:2 diet, is the most renowned intermittent fasting diet, also familiar as The Fast Diet, at the moment.

Michael Mosley, a British journalist, popularized it.

The 5:2 diet gets its name from the fact that 5 days in the week are allowed to eat normally, whereas the other 2 are limited to 500–600 calories per day.

This diet is more like a lifestyle than a diet because there are no restrictions on what foods you can eat, only when you will eat them.

This way of eating is easier to stick to for many people than a conventional calorie-restricted diet.

Everything that you need to understand about the 5:2 diet is explained below.

Diet review scorecard

- Overall rating: 3.96
- Weight loss 4.5
- Good nutrition 3.5
- Sustainability 4.75
- Total body health 2.25 for
- Nutritional value: 5 based
- on evidence 3.75

The End Result: The 5:2 diet is also an intermittent fasting protocol in which calorie intake is restricted to 500–600 calories twice a week. Fasting diets may be associated with a number of health benefits, but they may not be appropriate for everyone.

Chapter 6: The 5:2 diet

In this chapter, you will read everything you should know about the 5:2 diet. It will give you a total insight into this diet, what to do and what not to do.

It's actually quite simple to explain the 5:2 diet. You eat normally for five days a week and don't have to worry about calorie restriction.

Then you cut your calorie intake to 1/4 of your daily requirements on the other 2 days. This equates to around 500 calories a day for women & for men, it is 600 calories a day.

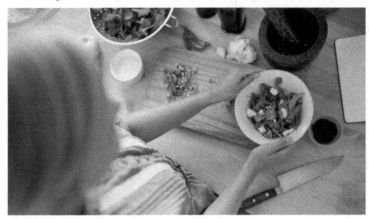

You can fast on any two days of the week that you want, as light as possible as there is at minimum 1 non-fasting day between.

Fasting on Mondays & Thursdays with 2 or 3 small meals, then eating normally for the remaining portion of the week, is a common method of organizing the week.

It's important to note that eating "normally" does not imply that you can eat whatever you want. If you eat junk food in excess, you are unlikely to lose weight but might gain weight.

You should eat as much as you would if you weren't fasting at all.

On the 5:2 diet, you eat normally five days a week and then limit your calorie intake to 500 to 600 calories the other 2 days.

6.1 Intermittent fasting has a number of health benefits.

There's very few research specifically on the 5:2 diet.

However, there are numerous studies on the health benefits of intermittent fasting in general.

Intermittent fasting has the advantage of being easier to stick to than constant calorie restriction, at least in some cases.

In addition, numerous studies have found that various types of intermittent fasting can significantly lower insulin levels.

According to one study, the 5:2 diet helped people lose weight in the same way that regular calorie limitation did. Furthermore, the diet was very successful in lowering insulin levels & improving insulin sensitivity.

Many other researchers have examined into the health impacts of customized alternate-day fasting that is similar to the 5:2 diet (though it is ultimately a 4:3 diet).

Insulin resistance, seasonal allergies, asthma, menopausal hot flashes, heart arrhythmias, and other conditions may be helped by the 4:3 diet.

When compared to a control group which ate normally, the group conducting 4:3 fasting showed significant improvements in both normalweight & overweight individuals.

The fasting community had after 12 weeks:

- Bodyweight was reduced by more than 5 kg (11 lbs.).
- Lost 7.7 lbs. (3.5 kg) of fat mass with no change.
- Triglyceride levels in the blood were reduced by 20%.
- LDL particle size has increased.
- CRP levels, an important inflammatory marker, are lower.
- Leptin levels were reduced by as much as 40%.

The 5:2 weight-loss diet

When done correctly, the 5:2 diet could be very effective for weight loss.

This is due to the 5:2 eating pattern's ability to help you eat fewer calories.

As a result, it is critical not to overeat on non-fasting days to reimburse for the fasting days.

If total calories are equal, intermittent fasting doesn't really cause the most weight loss than frequent calorie restriction.

Fasting protocols like the 5:2 diet, on the other hand, have shown a ton of potential in weight loss research:

- According to a recent study, adapted alternate-day fasting resulted in a weight loss of 3 to 8% over the course of 3 to 24 weeks (15).
- Participants in the same study lost 4 to 7% of their waist size, indicating that they lost a significant amount of damaging belly fat.
- When compared to traditional calorie restriction, intermittent fasting results in a much smaller loss of muscle mass.

When compound with exercises, such as strength training, or endurance intermittent fasting becomes even more effective.

If followed correctly, the 5:2 diet will help you lose weight quickly. It may aid in the reduction of belly fat as well as the preservation of muscle mass throughout weight loss.

6.2 On fasting days, what to eat

On fasting days, there are no rules about when to eat or what to eat it.

Some people work best when they start the day with a light breakfast, while others prefer to eat as late as possible.

In general, people follow one of 2 meal patterns:

1. **Three small meals:** Lunch, Breakfast, and dinner are the most common.

2. **There are only two slightly larger meals:** Dinner and lunch.

Because calorie intake is restricted (500 calories for women & 600 calories for men), it's important to make the most of your calorie budget.

Focus on foods that are nutritious, high in fiber, and high in protein to keep you full without consuming excessively.

On fast days, soups are really a great option. They may leave you feeling fuller than the same ingredients in their natural form or foods with the same calorie content, according to studies.

Here are some popular foods that could be eaten on a fast day:

- A large serving of vegetables
- Berries in natural yogurt
- Baked or boiled eggs
- Lean meat or grilled fish
- Rice made from cauliflower
- Soups
- Soups in a cup that are low in calories
- A cup of black coffee
- A cup of tea
- Water (still or sparkling)

On fasting days, there is no one-size-fits-all approach to eating. You'll need to experiment to see what works the best for you.

6.3
Delicious low-calorie meals

There are several sources on net that provide tasty 5:2 meal plans & recipes.

- They have a lot of low-calorie food suggestions.
- On the popular Fast Diet talk forum, you can find a wealth of facts and recipes.
- The 5:2 diet is also supported by a number of books and cookbooks, such as the best-selling books on the topic.

On the Internet, there are several meal plans & recipes for 500 600 calorie short days. It's a healthy thing to eat meals that are balanced, high in nutrients, & high in calcium.

6.4

What if you're sick or get an uncontrollable appetite

You should expect to feel very hungry within the 1st few days of your hard. It's also natural to feel less energized or sluggish than regular.

However, you'll be shocked by how easily the hunger subsides, particularly if you manage to keep yourself occupied with work and other errands.

In addition, after the 1st few fasts, most people notice that fast days get better.

If you're not used to fasting, it's a smart idea to have a little snack on hand for the first few fasts in case you get dizzy or sick.

However, if you consistently feel sick or faint during quick days, eat something and consult the doctor on whether you can proceed. Intermittent fasting isn't for everybody, and certain people can't stand it.

During the 1st few fasts, it's natural to feel hunger or lethargic. If you find yourself fainting or becoming sick sometimes, you should definitely abandon the diet.

Who can stay away from the 5:2 diet and intermittent fasting in general?

Intermittent fasting is really safe for those who are fit and well-nourished, but it is not for everybody.

Some individuals should totally stop food limits & fasting. There are some of them:

- People who have had an eating problem in the past.
- People who often suffer low blood sugar levels.
- Pregnant women, breastfeeding moms, adolescents, infants, and type 1 diabetics.

6.5

- Malnourished, underweight, or nutrition deficient people.
- Women that are unable to adopt or who are experiencing pregnancy problems.

Furthermore, certain women do not benefit as well from intermittent fasting as men do. Although adopting this eating trend, several people have confirmed that their menstrual periods have ended. As they switched to a daily diet, however, life returned to usual.

As a result, women should use caution before beginning some type of intermittent fasting, & should quit instantly if any negative results arise.

It is a simple and efficient way to shed pounds while still improving metabolic fitness.

It is much simpler to adhere to than a traditional calorie-restricted lifestyle for certain people.

The 5:2 plan is something to think about whether you choose to reduce weight or better your fitness.

Is Intermittent Fasting Successful in Increasing Metabolism?

Intermittent fasting (IF) is a form of eating that includes cycles of fasting followed by regular eating.

This eating pattern will help you lose weight, lower your risk of disease, and extend your life.

Some researchers also say that because of the metabolic benefits, it is a better way to reduce weight than traditional calorie restriction.

6.6
Weight Loss Can Be Achieved By Intermittent Fasting

Intermittent fasting is a quick, convenient, and reasonably easy-to-follow fat-loss strategy.

Intermittent fasting has been found in studies to be almost as efficient as, if not more effective than, conventional calorie restriction when it comes to weight reduction.

In reality, according to a 2014 study, intermittent fasting can help people lose 3 to 8% of their body mass in only 3 to 24 weeks.

Furthermore, a new study suggested that intermittent fasting could be a healthier weight-loss strategy for overweight & obese people than lowcalorie diets.

Surprisingly, this way of eating can even be beneficial to your metabolism and overall health.

Intermittent fasting can be done in a variety of forms. The 5:2 diet, that includes fasting 2 days a week, is followed by certain individuals. Others follow the 16/8 approach or alternate-day fasting.

If you want to learn all about intermittent fasting, check out this comprehensive tutorial for beginners.

An intermittent diet is a great way to lose weight. It will even help you lose weight and increase your metabolic fitness.

Chapter 7: Fundamentals of Intermittent Fasting

Hormones are chemical messengers that help us communicate with one another. They migrate around the body to help complex processes like development & metabolism run smoothly.

They too play an important part in weight management. This is due to the fact that they have a significant impact on one's hunger, the number of calories you consume, and the amount of fat you accumulate or burn.

Enhancements in the stability of certain fat-burning hormones have been attributed to intermittent fasting. This might render it an effective weightloss tool.

7.1
Insulin

Insulin is a hormone that plays a key role in fat metabolism. Which tells the body to accumulate fat & prevents it from being broken down.

Having chronically elevated insulin levels will make losing weight even more difficult. Obesity, type 2 diabetes, cardiac failure, and cancer have also been attributed to high insulin levels.

Intermittent fasting has been found to be almost as good at reducing insulin levels as calorie-restricted diets.

In reality, this eating pattern can lower fasting blood glucose by 20 to 31%.

7.2

Human growth hormone

Fasting may induce an increase in human growth hormone levels in the blood, which is an essential hormone for fat loss.

Fasting has been found to raise elements of social growth hormone in men by up to five-fold in several research.

Increased amounts of growth hormone in the blood stimulate fat burning while both preserving muscle mass & providing other advantages.

Women, on the other hand, don't necessarily reap the same gains from fasting as males, and it's unclear if women would see the same increase in people's growth hormone.

7.3
Norepinephrine

The "fight - or - flight" reaction is aided by norepinephrine, a tension hormone that increases alertness and concentration.

It has a host of other impacts on the body, one of which is inducing fatty acid release in your fat cells.

Increased norepinephrine levels usually result in more fat being accessible for the body to burn.

The level of norepinephrine in one's bloodstream increases as you quick.

Fasting can help lower insulin levels while still increasing the number of human growth hormones & norepinephrine in the blood. These improvements will make it easier for you to burn fat and lose weight.

7.4
Short-term fasts boost metabolism by up to 14%

Many people assume that missing meals causes the body to adjust by slowing down your metabolism in order to save resources.

It's well known that going without food for long stretches of time will trigger a decrease in metabolism.

Short-term fasting, on the other hand, has been found to speed up rather than slow down your metabolism.

A three-day quick improved the metabolism of 11 healthy men by 14 percent, according to one report.

This spike is believed to be attributed to an increase in the fat-burning hormone norepinephrine.

Fasting for a brief amount of time will help to speed up one's metabolism. Fasting for lengthy periods of time, on the other hand, can have the reverse impact.

Intermittent fasting reduces metabolism well below calorie restriction in a continuous basis

Your metabolic ratio decreases when you drop weight. Most of this is due to the fact that gaining weight results in muscle weakness, & muscle tissue consumes calories all day long.

However, the drop in metabolic rate associated with weight loss isn't always due to a loss in muscle mass.

7.5

Long-term calorie restriction will trigger your metabolism to decrease as your body enters "starvation mode" (also known as "adaptive thermogenesis"). As normal protection against hunger, the body does this to save resources.

This was shown significantly in a survey of individuals who shed significant sums of weight when competing on the TV show The Biggest Loser.

To shed a lot of weight, the participants adopted a calorie-limited diet & did a lot of exercises.

The majority of them had recovered almost all of the weight one had lost six years later, according to the report. Their metabolic speeds, on the other hand, had not increased and stayed about 500 calories less than would be expected for your body size.

Related findings have been observed in several experiments looking at the impact of calorie restriction for weight reduction. Weight loss will trigger a reduction in metabolism that can cost 100 of calories a day.

This proves that "starvation mode" exists, and it can help to understand why so many people that lose weight gain it back.

Given the short-term effect of fasting in hormones, intermittent fasting can help to offset the metabolic slowdown induced through long-term calorie restriction.

Over the course of 22 days, a limited sample found that gaining weight through an alternative fasting diet would not decrease metabolism.

However, no high-quality study on the long-term impact to intermittent fasting diets in metabolic rate is currently possible.

According to one small report, intermittent fasting can help to prevent the decrease in metabolism that comes with weight loss. More investigation is needed.

7.6 Intermittent fasting aids in the preservation of muscle mass

Muscle is a metabolism tissue that aids in maintaining a high metabolic rate. And while you're at rest, this makes you eat more calories. When individuals lose weight, they usually lose both fat & muscle.

Because of its role on fat-burning hormones, intermittent fasting has been believed to maintain muscle mass more than calorie restriction.

Even if you're losing weight, the rise in growth hormone shown through fasting will help you keep your muscle mass.

Intermittent fasting was shown to be more efficient than a conventional low-calorie diet at maintaining muscle throughout weight loss in a 2011 study.

The findings, however, have also been mixed. Intermittent fasting and prolonged calorie restriction have a comparable impact on lean body fat, according to a recent study.

After eight weeks, a new report showed little disparity in lean body mass between those who were fasting & others who were under constant calorie restriction. Those in the fasting category, on the other hand, had lost fewer lean body fat after 24 weeks.

To figure out intermittent fasting is much more successful at maintaining lean body mass, larger and longer trials are required.

Intermittent fasting can help you lose weight by reducing the amount of weight you lose. However, the evidence is contradictory.

Recommended foods & tips

While the 16:8 schedule for intermittent fasting does not dictate which foods to consume and which to skip, focusing on healthy nutrition and limiting or excluding junk foods is helpful. Excessive intake of unhealthy foods may lead to weight gain & contribute to disease.

A well-balanced diet emphasizes:

- Organic, frozen, or canned fruits & vegetables (in water) Quinoa,
- peas, brown rice, and barley are all whole grains.
- Pork, fish, lentils, beans, tofu, almonds, seeds, low-fat cottage cheese, & eggs are also good sources of lean protein.
- Oily fish, olives, coconuts, olive oil, avocados, almonds, and seeds are also good sources of healthy fats.

Fiber-rich foods like vegetables, fruits, and whole grains will make an individual feel complete and happy. Satiety may also be enhanced by eating healthy fats & proteins.

For those adopting the 16:8 schedule for intermittent fasting diet, beverages may help with satiety. Since people sometimes confuse appetite with hunger, drinking water during the day will help you consume less calories.

During the 16-hour fasting time, the 16:8 diet schedule allows you to consume calorie-free beverages like water & unsweetened tea & coffee. To stop dehydration, it's important to drink water on a daily basis.

Tips

People who adopt these tips can find it much easier to adhere to the 16:8 diet:

- During fasting time, sip cinnamon herbal tea to reduce your appetite.
- Drinking plenty of water during the day
- Viewing less to avoid being exposed to pictures of food that can arouse a desire to eat
- Exercising just before or after a meal, since exercise will make you hungry.
- While preparing meals, being careful of what you're doing
- Meditating through the fasting time to alleviate hunger pangs

Briefly, below are the seven most important suggestions:

- Drink plenty of water.
- Keep yourself occupied.
- Get a cup of coffee or tea.
- Survive the hunger pangs.
- Try extended fasting (such as 16:8) for a month to see if it's right for you.
- In between fasting hours, eat a low-carb diet. This suppresses appetite and facilitates intermittent fasting.

It can also have a greater impact on weight loss and type 2 diabetes reversal, among other things.

- Don't overeat after a fast.

7.7 Risks and Side Effects

Intermittent fasting at a 16:8 ratio has certain complications and side effects. As a consequence, the strategy isn't enough for everybody.

- In the early phases of the program, hunger, fatigue, and tiredness are possible side effects & threats.
- Due to extreme appetite, overeating, or consuming unhealthful items during the 8-hrs. eating window
- Overeating causes heartburn or reflux.

Women can benefit less from intermittent fasting than men. Intermittent fasting has been shown in animal studies to have a detrimental impact on female fertility.

Intermittent fasting can be avoided for those who have a history of maladaptive feeding. Fasting is a contributing factor for eating disorders, according to the National Eating Disorders Association.

Someone with a history of anxiety or depression may still find the 16:8 strategy unsuitable. According to certain studies, calorie restriction for a brief period of time may help with depression, however prolonged calorie restriction may have the reverse impact. To fully comprehend the consequences of these results, further study is needed.

Many that are nursing, breastfeeding, or attempting to conceive can avoid 16:8 intermittent fasting.

According to the National Institute on Aging, there is inadequate evidence to suggest some fasting diets, particularly for older adults.

People who choose to pursue the 16:8 approach or other forms of intermittent fasting must first consult their doctor, particularly if they are on certain drugs or have any of the following conditions:

- A pre-existing medical disorder, such as asthma or high blood pressure
- A prevalence of eating disorders
- A family history of psychiatric illness

Anyone who has reservations about the diet or is experiencing negative symptoms should see a physician.

Isn't intermittent fasting going to make us hungry?

It's unlikely. Which is the most prevalent misconception concerning intermittent fasting, & it is usually untrue.

In reality, some research suggests that intermittent fasting can boost overall body composition by raising the basal metabolic ratio (at least initially).

Is it possible to work out when fasting?

Yes, really. When fasting, you will manage to do all of your normal tasks, including exercise.

You don't need to consume much until working out to provide enough juice.

Instead, the body can use surplus resources (such as body fat) as a source of energy.

However, eating before longs-duration aerobic exercise can help you perform better.

While fasting, it's often important to consume water & replenish sodium around exercise. If you're playing, you should be aware of this.

What are the potential negative consequences?

Intermittent fasting may have a variety of negative consequences.

If you come across them, here's what you can do:

- The most frequent side effect to intermittent fasting is hunger. If you're still on a keto diet or low-carb, high-fat diet, this might not be a problem.

- Constipation is a natural occurrence. Fewer coming in equals less leaving. Bear in mind that this is a natural reaction to consuming less. If you have extreme bloating or stomach pain, it isn't a cause for alarm and shouldn't be treated. If necessary, magnesium supplements or standard laxatives may be used.

- Headaches are normal and usually subside after the 1ts few fasts.

Adding a pinch of salt to your diet will help you avoid headaches.

- If their stomach gurgles, mineral water can aid.

- Dizziness, heartburn, and muscle cramps are also potential side effects.

The refeeding condition is a more severe side effect. Fortunately, this is uncommon, occurring only during prolonged fasts (5 to10 days or longer) while one is malnourished.

Since the majority of these adverse effects are manageable, you do not need to break yours soon. However, you can break your fast if you are truly sick, severely tired, excessively dizzy, or have any serious symptoms.

Just try to take it gently before breaking it and to put fluids and salt first. Of course, unless the signs continue, you can see a doctor right away.

Strong side effects, on the other hand, are very uncommon, particularly if you stay hydrated & take electrolytes. **Why would our blood sugar rise during fast?**

Although not everyone experiences this, it may happen as a result of hormone shifts that arise throughout intermittent fasting. Sugar is generated by your body to provide energy to your system. This is a variant of the dawn effect, and it is generally unproblematic as soon as blood sugar levels do not rise during the day.

How can you deal with hunger?

The most critical thing to remember is that hunger is a wave that comes and goes. Many people fear that hunger will intensify before it becomes unbearable during intermittent fasting, but this is seldom the case.

Hunger, on the other hand, arrives in waves. It would usually pass if you just forget it & drink a cup of coffee or tea.

During long fasts, hunger levels often rise on the 2nd day. After that, it eventually fades, and by day 3 or 4, many people mention no longer feeling hungry.

Fat is also the source of energy for the body. And other words, the body is no longer starving when it is 'eating' its very own fat with breakfast, lunch, and dinner. Find out more.

Isn't intermittent fasting going to make you lose muscle?

This is dependent on the individual & the length of the short. The body breaks glycogen into glucose to energy during fasting. Following that, the body grows fat breakdown in order to supply nutrition.

Excess amino acids (protein building blocks) are often used for nutrition, although the body should not burn its very own muscle until it is absolutely necessary.

However, some research suggests that leaner people are more likely to lose lean body fat and even have a lower metabolic rate. However, it seems that this is lesser of a problem in overweight people. **Is intermittent fasting suitable for senior citizens?**

Before you jump into this new eating pattern, make sure you're aware of the dangers.

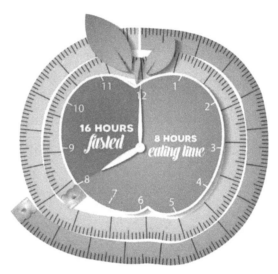

Intermittent fasting is a common feeding technique that is being researched in labs and used in kitchens all over the United States. And it isn't just a fad. Restricting the calorie intake or mealtimes can have a number of advantages, including weight reduction and a lower chance of multiple diseases. However, there isn't any research on the impact of intermittent fasting on the well-being of older people.

Risks that may occur

Although intermittent fasting has shown potential, there isn't enough research to support its effects or how it can impact older adults. Small numbers of middle-aged or young people have been studied in humans for only a brief interval of time.

However, we do know that intermittent fasting may be dangerous in certain situations. "I'd be worried if you're still marginal in terms of body weight," McManus says, "because losing so much weight will damage the muscles, overall immune system, & energy level."

Another problem, according to Dr. Suzanne Salamon, associate head of gerontology of Harvard-affiliated Beth Israel Deaconess Medical Center: "Fasting can be difficult for people who need to take their drugs with food to prevent discomfort or stomach irritation. Additionally, people who take cardiac or blood pressure drugs might be more susceptible to harmful potassium & sodium imbalances while fasting."

If you do have diabetes & require food at certain hours, or if you take blood-sugar-lowering drugs, intermittent fasting can be dangerous.

7.8 Pitfalls to Avoid

For anyone who consumes every few hours, this form of diet will be impossible (e.g., snacks b/w meals, grazes). That may also be inappropriate for people with diseases including diabetes, which necessitate eating at frequent periods due to metabolic shifts induced by their drugs. If food is brought back after a long time of food scarcity or semi-starvation, one is at risk of overeating, which can lead to risky habits including an intensified focus on food.

Intermittent fasting can be avoided for those who have the following conditions:

- Diabetes
- Eating conditions including excessive self-restriction (anorexia nervosa or bulimia nervosa)
- Treatment that necessitates food consumption
- Teens in active development stages Pregnancy
- and breastfeeding

Do you really want to give it a shot?

Speak to your doctor if you're thinking of attempting intermittent fasting, particularly if you already have a health problem like diabetes or heart disease.

McManus suggests off slowly with the diet. "Over a span of many months, gradually reduce the window of time for feeding," she suggests.

Often, follow the doctor's instructions for taking your medications. Dr. Alexander Soukas, an endocrinologist & molecular geneticist at General Hospital Harvard-affiliated Massachusetts, claims that taking drugs doesn't break the hard, and neither does drinking calorie-free beverages like water or black coffee.

What if you need food in addition to your medication? "You might want to try a tweaked quick. I believe it will also be beneficial to those that are overweight "According to Dr. Salamon."Just hammer out a prescription with one's doctor that would support your life without putting it at risk."

Sticking a Toe in the Water

There are ways to utilize some of the pillars of IF to raise the GH without triggering cortisol havoc.

- Quick for at least 12 hours without eating. Remember the change from dinner to breakfast.
- If you're not sleepy, put off eating for a bit while. Enable for a 14-hour break b/w meals.
- Feed-in between meals as little as possible. Avoid eating tiny meals often during the day. Eat a high-protein breakfast, lunch, and dinner without snacking in between.
- A smoothie is an easy-to-digest breakfast choice. Increase the amount of liquid-based meals to two a day (smoothie or soup).
- Restrict the post-workout feeding to whey protein, which has been shown to improve muscle protein composition time after time. Carbohydrate consumption may reduce GH output.
- If you've overindulged the night before, fasting and running at a high pace will help you lose weight and overweight.
- If you train moderately for less than an hrs. a day, nothing relates to you. If you're a high-intensity athlete who has to rebound from 1 bout of exercise in order to conduct a second later another workout or in the day the next day, you can need more carbohydrate-based food to avoid depleting your stocks.

Chapter 8: Fasting- Tips & Tricks for Woman

In this chapter, you will go through the process of fasting. How to live your daily life during fasting and all the techniques of fasting for a woman.

8.1 What is the best way to end a fast?

Gently, please. You will need to be gentler as the quick advances.

A stomach ache may be caused by eating too big of food after fasting (a big mistake that we've all made, including yourself). Although this is not a dangerous condition, most people soon learn to eat as fully as possible after such a short.

Isn't it important to consume breakfast every day?

Certainly not. It's an old myth founded on conjecture & statistics that struggles to stand up when put to the test.

Through missing breakfast, the body has much time to burn calories for energy. Since hunger is at its lowest as in the morning, skipping breakfast and breaking the fast later throughout the day could be the easiest option.

- Skipping morning meals doesn't imply that you can eat more.
- New York Times: Breakfast isn't particularly magical.

8.2 Fasting for woman

However, there are several variations. Fasting is not recommended for women who already are underweight, pregnant, or breastfeeding.

In addition, women who are trying to conceive should be mindful that intermittent fasting may raise the risk of unstable menses and reduce the chances of pregnancy, especially in athletic women with a low body fat percentage.

Besides, there is no compelling justification for women to refrain from fasting.

Intermittent fasting will trigger complications for both men and women. Women do not often get the outcome they want, but men do as well.

According to studies, women & men that fast lose equal amounts of weight.

Isn't fasting the same as calorie reduction?

No, it is not the case. Fasting will help you waste less time consuming by addressing the issue of "what to feed."

The issue of "whether & how much to eat" is answered by calorie restriction. They are two related topics which shouldn't be mistaken.

Fasting can help you lose weight, but the advantages go well beyond that.

Would you be able to lose weight?

Almost definitely. When one needs to lose weight, one can almost certainly lose weight if ones don't feed.

Of note, it is theoretically probable to consume more during fasting, negating the weight loss. However, surveys indicate that other people consume considerably less in total.

Intermittent fasting is known as "the ancient mystery to weight loss" and it is one of the most effective nutritional techniques for weight loss, but it has long been overlooked by physicians and dietitians.

8.3 We've found that intermittent fasting has made our life easier and happier

We were allowed to consume the things we liked and much of our daily meals, but only for eight to ten hours at a time.

We started an intermittent fasting diet earlier this year at the suggestion of doctor friends & after reading a few famous novels. The fundamentals are that we could consume any foods we chose and much of our daily meals, but just for eight to ten hours at a time. Aside from that, you'd drink just water, tea, & black coffee.

Intermittent fasting, often known as a time-restricted diet, proponents say, might help us lose weight, which is still a worthy objective. It will also give your stomach a much-needed escape from food production, increase concentration, and reduce inflammation on a regular basis. It could also help us live longer in the long run.

We'll confess that the phrase "intermittent fasting" intimidated me. Dr. Jason Fung, creator of "The Obesity Code," told us, though, that it will be easy to integrate into one's everyday life.

"Anytime you don't feed for more than 4 hrs. is fasting," he clarified. "Many people consume because they'll have to rather than because they like what they are consuming. If you don't want to consume the sandwich, don't. Your body will do as it is designed to do: it will lose one's body fat. That's why you have it in your bag."

In other terms, by voluntarily refusing yourself food for lengthy stretches of time throughout the day, your body will turn from burning sugar to burning fat as a source of energy.

Two reasons lead us to conclude that we would be willing to adhere to an intermittent fasting protocol. To begin with, we have Type one diabetes, which necessitates deliberate feeding. For the majority of our life, we've spent our days calculating whether we should or might not eat in the moment, evaluating the advantages and disadvantages of different foods when taking into consideration factors like calories, sugar, and fiber. If we are very careful, you will get some protein as well. We have to remember more the more we feed.

Second, we did the Whole30 program last year, which required us to avoid much of the foods one enjoys: no eggs, no wheat or grains, no soy, no sugar, and no alcohol. And items that we considered to be safe, such as chickpeas, were prohibited. We liked the diet because of its specific guidelines, but any time we tried to adhere to it within the first 30 days, one may struggle. Travel or out-of-town dinners will come up. It was as adaptable as Cersei, the Iron Throne's queen.

Choosing how long to fast was the first phase in the intermittent fasting path. Diet research is only in the early stages, and the time ranges within which you're required to consume range from eight to ten hours. According to some studies, shorter is easier, so we went for eight hours, starting at 11 a.m. and ending at 7 p.m. we promised that after dinner, we would just drink herbal tea. We had been a late-night snack for decades. Then we went to the store and prayed while purchasing some fancy teas.

The rest was simple once you settled on the timetable. You may settle into a comfortable routine that consisted of 2 meals a day & a little lunch in between. Salads, eggs, pork, fruits, milk, nuts and fruit, and a cookie or the odd square of dark chocolate were the mainstays of your diet.

Unlike the Whole thirty, time-restricted dining gave us the flexibility we needed. We may drink that bottle of champagne, consume that wedge of cheese, & return to the love for chickpeas, our spirit animal legume. The strength about this diet is that it has concentrated on what we ate instead of what we ate. We could consume anything we wanted, and as much as we wanted, during our nonfasting hours. While we were still conscious, being out of calorie counting was a welcome relief.

Intermittent fasting often gave us a more Zen-like attitude to the waking hours, which we quickly realized was something we really needed. And our emotional burden, the one we have from dealing with diabetes went "poof" when we stopped consuming three or 5 meals a day.

Dr. Jake Kushner, a pediatric endocrinologist who used to work at Baylor College but now works at McNair Interest, a private equity company, was sympathetic to the plight. "People with diabetes will slay it very well, but they are to get up tomorrow & slay it all over again," he said, which we understood all too well from the own Type 1 diabetes experience.

Dr. Kushner challenged us to think of an amount between 1 & 10. "Your cognitive load is calculated by adding up the time one spent worrying about diabetes. The first is that we are aware that we have it, but you are unconcerned with it. The number ten means that you just care of insulin and that it has taken over one's thoughts." It is based on a history of eating with Form 1, I offered him the number 7. However, as a result of introducing intermittent fasting, the amount of cognitive load was gradually declining.

We took less insulin because we were just consuming two meals a day. We will happily work on our laptop, drink coffee, and forget blood sugar levels for the 1st half of the day. Though we had hunger pangs at first, they subsided quickly, & we found ourselves staying hrs. Longer on several days before eating the first meal. We'll confess that we enjoyed having complete power of the body.

Though intermittent fasting is simple to implement, you were far from perfect, and you can found ourselves dropping off the wagon most times, particularly on days when you ate out with friends, making yourself wonder if you were undoing any possible gains. Dr. Satchin Panda, the author of "The Circadian Code" & a researcher only at Salk Institute, addressed the query.

On our days off, Dr. Panda told us that we shall continue to earn benefits. The mice in his experiments, like me, were given weekends off & were able to consume as much as they wanted. "However, the bulk of the advantages of time-restricted feeding were maintained," he clarified. "These involve decreased body weight, body fat, and cholesterol, as well as improved carbohydrate regulation, liver fat reduction, greater mobility, and improved muscle coordination."

We did note that we were sleeping well. "Not wanting food in the stomach aids us in getting a good night's sleep," Dr. Panda said. "If you do timerestricted feeding, your sleeping drive will improve, and your sleeping would be much better," he said, but the mice he observed were unable to tell him this.

Dr. Panda claimed that heart failure is the leading cause of death worldwide and that tests have found that fasting, which also occurs in dietary restriction, improves the life expectancy of even healthier individuals. Fasting can also help to suppress tumor growth and avoid outbreaks of breast cancer & other cancers, according to reports.

Dr. Panda said, "What we're seeing is the 1st wave of this study." "The second phase will arrive in 2020, where we will see more thorough disease research. We'll still look at harmful side effects, but just because there aren't any of these retrospective trials doesn't suggest they don't exist."

What we've found is that when we fast, our mental clarity increases and blood sugar levels are less unpredictable — a win-win scenario for everybody. Then, when we're asleep, blood sugar stays in a healthier, safe range, out of the normal food-related ups and downs.

We are still keeping an eye on our mental figure, which Dr. Kushner advised us to keep a note of. The emotional amount looked like a 3 or 4 on a strong day of intermittent fasting.

However, another of Dr. Kushner's ideas springs to mind. "At any point, you can experiment with the keto diet," he said, pointing to a diet in which net carbs are limited to fewer than 20 gm per day. Animal proteins, dairy, fats, and very particular low-carb veggies like broccoli, cauliflower, and zucchini are the diet's mainstays. "Keto people claim two," he said. "What occurs is that the glucose difference in your blood stops. You recover your life. You get the time to worry about other things. People with Type 1 lose their capacity to be human, special, and to care of other things."

But, after discovering the joys of extended fasting, one might not able to follow yet another set of eating guidelines. Even next year.

Chapter 9: The Benefits and Drawbacks to Exercising Whilst On a Fast

Whether you're new to intermittent fasting (IF) or fasting for some cause and want to start working out, there are a few pros & cons to remember when choosing to exercise when fasted.

According to certain studies, exercise while fasting changes muscle biochemistry & metabolism, which are related to insulin sensitivity and blood sugar level control.

Eating and exercising right afterward, until digestion or absorption, has often been shown to be beneficial. This is especially significant for people who have types 2 diabetes or suffer from metabolic syndrome.

One advantage of fasting, according to Chelsea Amengual, MS, RD, who is the manager of Fitness Programming and Nutrition of Virtual Health Partners, is that your accumulated carbs, identified as glycogen, are more definitely exhausted, meaning you'll be burning more fat to fuel your exercise.

Does the thought of burning more fat sound appealing? There is a drawback to the fasting conditions cardio trend that you should be aware of before jumping on board.

It's likely that if you exercise when fasted, the body can start breaking off muscle and use protein as food, according to Amengual. "Plus, you're more apt to touch a wall," she continues, "which ensures you'll have less stamina and won't be capable of working out as much or do as well."

Intermittent fasting and long-term workout, according to Priya Khorana, EdD, a diet instructor at Columbia University, aren't suitable. "The body depletes itself from calories and electricity, which may cause the metabolism to slow down," she continues.

9.1 Exercise whilst one is fasting

- If you fast for an extended period of time, your metabolism can slow down.
- You might not be willing to offer the full effort during workouts.
- You can lose fat or just be able to retain muscle mass rather than develop it.

Getting a good workout when fasting is possible.

If you choose to pursue intermittent fasting while continuing to exercise, there are a few items you could do to make the work out more successful.

1. Consider the pacing

When it comes to getting the work out more successful when fasting, registered dietician Christopher Shuff says there are three things to consider: whether you can exercise before, after, or after the fueling window.

The 16:8 protocol is a common IF form. The definition involves eating everything during an 8-hour fueling timeframe before fasting for 16 hours.

"Exercising out before the window is perfect for someone who does well during work out on an empty stomach, and working out during the window is better for someone who doesn't want to exercise on an empty belly but needs to take advantage of post-workout nutrition," he says. During is the safest choice for success and regeneration, according to Shuff.

He continues, "After the window was for those who want to work out after fueling but don't have time to do so during the feeding window."

2. Determine the kind of exercise you can do depending on your macros

Lynda Lippin, a licensed personal trainer & Master Pilate's instructor, says it's essential to give attention to the macronutrients you ingest the day before and after you work out.

Power exercises, for example, necessitate further carbs on the day of the exercise, while [high-intensity interval training] cardio/HIIT may be performed on a lower carbs day, she describes.

3. To develop or sustain strength, eat the right foods during the exercise

According to Dr. Niket Sonpal, the easiest way to combine IF and fitness is to schedule your exercises during your eating cycles so that your nutrition rates are at their highest.

"It's also essential to your body to also have proteins after a heavy lifting exercise to help in regeneration," he continues.

Following some strength exercise, Amengual recommends eating carbs and around 20 grams of protein within 30 minutes of the workout.

9.2 Work out comfortably while fasting

Any weight reduction or fitness program's effectiveness is determined by how secure it is to maintain over time. Keep in a safe place if your overarching target is to lose body fat & preserve your health level when doing IF. Here are few professional suggestions to assist you in doing so. **Closely follow the mild- to high-intensity exercise with a meal**

This is when the importance of meal planning falls into action. It's crucial, according to Khorana, to eat prior to a low- or high-intensity exercise. As a consequence, the body may have some glycogen supplies to draw from to power your exercise. **Keep yourself hydrated.**

It's important to note that fasting does not imply dehydration, according to Sonpal. In reality, he advises drinking more water when fasting.

Maintain a balanced electrolyte level

Coconut water, according to Sonpal, is a healthy low-calorie hydration source. It claims that it replenishes electrolytes, is low in calories, and tastes nice. Stop consuming too much Gatorade or athletic beverages since they are rich in sugar.

Maintain a low level of severity & length

Take a rest if you light-headed or feel dizzy after working yourself so hard. It's important to pay attention to the body.

Think of the kind of quick you'll be doing

If you're doing a 24-hrs sporadic easy, Lippin suggests doing low-intensity exercises like:

- Jogging
- Yoga for relaxing
- Pilates (gentle)

However, since most of the 16 hrs. Fasting window is spent in the evening, sleeping, and early in the morning if you're doing the 16:8 fasting, keeping to a certain form of work out isn't as essential.

Pay attention to the body

When exercising during IF, the most important thing to remember is to respond to your body.

"If you tend to feel tired or dizzy, it's likely that you have dehydrated or are low blood sugar," Amengual says. If that's the case, she suggests beginning with an electrolyte-carbohydrate drink and then consuming a well-balanced lunch.

Although exercising & intermittent fasting can be beneficial to certain individuals, others may be uncomfortable exercising at all while fasting.

Before initiating any food or fitness regimen, contact the healthcare or doctor professional.

On October 26, 2018, a surgical examination was completed.

9.3 Possibility to lose weight quicker if you work out with an empty stomach

Experts weigh in on the benefits of fasted cardio.

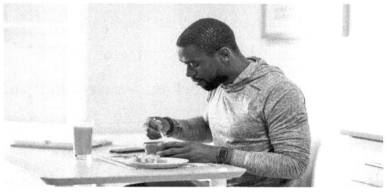

Have you ever been advised to exercise with an empty stomach? Cardio is done, or fasted cardio before or after feeding, is a common subject in the health and diet community.

There are proponents and opponents, as with many wellness phenomena. Some people swear it's an easy and successful way to lose weight, whilst others think it's a waste of time & money.

Fasted cardio doesn't often imply that you're doing an intermittent fast plan. It may be as straightforward as heading on a run 1st thing in the morning and then having breakfast.

The benefits and drawbacks of fasted cardio were discussed with three health and diet experts. This is what they have to suggest about it.

1. Give it a shot: Fasted cardio can help you burn calories

In weight loss and exercise circles, upright cycle or hitting the treadmill for a workout session while eating is popular. The promise of burning extra fat is always the key motivator. So how does it work in practice?

Emmie Satrazemis, RD, CSSD, certified board and certified sports nutritionist & nutrition director at Trifecta, says, "Not getting extra calories or pre-workout snack food on hand from a recent meal or forces the body to focus on stored fuel, that happens to be glycogen & stored fat."

She points to minor studies

Exercising in the morning while fasting for 8-12 hrs. through sleep, according to a reliable source, will help you burn up to 20% more fat. Even so, there are studies that indicate it has little impact on total fat.

2. Skip It: Eating before a cardio workout is essential if you are trying to burn more fat

However, there is a distinction to be established between acquiring muscle mass & retaining muscle mass.

"As long as you eat enough protein and use one's muscles, research indicates that muscle mass is reasonably well covered, even in a calorie deficit," Satrazemis explains.

That's because amino acids aren't as attractive as stored carbohydrates and fat while your body is searching for food. Satrazemis, on the other side, argues that the supply of rapid energy is minimal, and that exercising too hard for far too long when fasting can cause one to run out of energy or begin to break down more muscle.

She also believes that eating after such a workout helps you to replenish such stocks as well as fix the muscle loss that happened during the workout.

3. Give It a Shot: People like The Way Fasted Cardio Makes One Body Sound

This explanation can seem self-evident, but it's not unusual to ask why we do stuff, even though they make you happy. As a result, Satrazemis believes that the choice to pursue fasted cardio is a personal one. "Some people like to exercise on an empty stomach, whilst others do best while they eat," she explains.

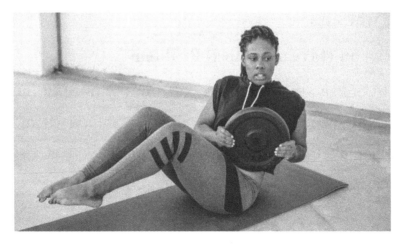

4. Don't Do It: Things That Involve a Lot of Strength and Pace Can Be Undertaken With Food in the Stomach

As per David Chesworth, which is an ACSM-certified personal trainer, if you intend on doing an exercise that requires high amounts of strength or pace, you can eat before doing certain exercises.

He explains why glucose is the best fuel for strength and pace operations since it is the fastest type of energy. "The physiology does not usually provide the optimal tools for this form of exercise in a fasted state," Chesworth notes. As a result, if you want to get quick and strong, he recommends training after you've eaten.

5. Give It A Shot: If you're Dealing with Gi Issues, Quick Exercise Can Be Beneficial

If you eat even a snack or a meal before performing the exercise, you can feel nauseous throughout your workout. "This is particularly true in the morning, as well as with high fat & high fiber foods," Satrazemis says.

If you can't afford a bigger meal or don't have at least 2 hours to process it, you could be best served eating anything with a simple energy supply — or doing exercise when fasted.

6. Don't Do It: You Have a Medical Problem

You must be in outstanding shape to perform cardio in a fasted condition. You can also remember health issues like low blood sugar or low blood pressure, which may induce dizziness and place you at risk for injuries, according to Satrazemis.

9.4 Tools for performing fasted cardio in a rush

If you wish to attempt fasted cardio, keep the following guidelines in mind to ensure your safety:

- Should not workout for longer than 60 mins without resting.
- Choose exercises that are mild or low-intensity.
- Drinking water is a part of quick cardio, so remain hydrated.
- Keep in mind that your overall lifestyle, particularly your diet, has a greater impact on your weight loss or gain than the frequency of your workouts.

Pay attention to the health & do what feels right. If you're unsure about whether or not you can perform fasted cardio, seek advice from a personal trainer, licensed dietician, or doctor.

Chapter 10: Learning What Is Wrong and How to Make It Right!

We include items that we feel would be helpful to our readers. Let's keep the truth straight, not just for our own sake, but also because we need them to eat well.

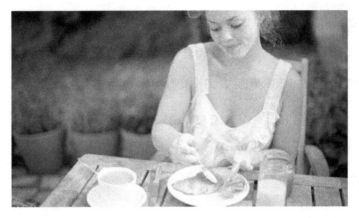

The intermittent fasting craze arrived like a lion, and it turns out that we got a couple of items wrong in the process.

We sat with Dr. Valter Longo, (director of the University of Southern California's Longevity Institute and creator of "The Longevity Diet,") to unpack the hysteria and isolate reality from sensationalism.

Here's his opinion upon on intermittent fasting craze, as well as several pointers to help you better grasp the idea and put it into practice.

10.1
Our Terminology is incorrect

For starters, intermittent fasting does not have the same sense as we assume it does. When we discuss Leangains' 16:8 regimen or the 5:2 plan as IF processes, we're just talking about time-restricted eating (TRF).

Dr. Longo notes that the acronym IF "represents a troublesome way because it encourages individuals to improvise and select and choose times of fasting that extend from 12 hrs. to weeks, providing the appearance that... every 'abstention from food' is equal or comparable, and both have health benefits" in his book "The Longevity Diet."

Dr. Longo's recommendation is to "keep using the right terminology" to get in the best attitude. If you go without food for less than 24 hours, you are not fasting. Time-restricted feeding is the right concept.

10.2

Going to extremes isn't necessarily the only option

On a daily basis, abstain for 16-24 hrs. between feeding sessions, according to common IF advice online. Dr. Longo, on the other side, suggests a window of the feeding of twelve hrs. a day for optimum fitness.

Although the dietary psychology of intermittent fasting obviously appeals to certain individuals, especially when practiced for a brief period of time, traditional IF advice can pose health risks.

If you just feed for four or 6 hrs. a day, "then you tend to see gallstone forming [and] raise the risk that you'll get your gallbladder removed," says Dr. Longo.

Longer cycles between meals, regardless of weight, have been found in studies to raise the risk of gallstone development in women.

Although no precise link has been established, studies show that people who miss breakfast have a higher risk of cardiovascular disease, cancer, and death.

Extremely restricted feeding windows & alternate-day fasting may also raise the likelihood of cardiovascular disease, while a report on flies showed that 12-hour TRF decreased age-related cardiac decline.

On the other side, "if you consume 15 hrs. per day or more, it begins to be correlated with metabolic conditions, sleep disturbances, and so on," according to Longo.

Dr. Longo's recommendation is to eat for 12 hrs. and then fast for another 12. To avoid negative health consequences, stick to this normal feeding regimen as near as possible.

10.3

Time-restricted eating is a long-term behavioral improvement, not a fast remedy

It's tempting to believe in the hype of radical food fast fixes, but you hardly learn of someone living to be 100 when following a fad diet.

One of the five foundations that Dr. Longo uses to help his longevity study is centenarian studies. In long-term implications and practicality, they often show what clinical trials cannot.

Dr. Longo advises dropping back to two meals and a snack per day instead of his normal three meals & a couple of snacks.

Other important procedures in high-longevity areas include:

- adopting a pescatarian lifestyle (no meat, only seafood)
- eating a modest level of protein before the age of 65
- limiting sugar consumption

Advice from Dr. Longo: We could learn a lot from our elders' eating habits, particularly the elderly. They are walking examples of what encourages good health & long lives.

Does it assist you in living longer?

Scientific Americans looked through the study on IF and discovered that it may aid with survival, but the proof isn't definitive.

Finding the best feeding time doesn't have to be difficult

What is Dr. Longo's 12-hour regular feeding window? It's likely that you're still doing that.

You're there in a sweet spot if you grab breakfast around 8:00 pm, lunch at midday, then stop feeding until dinner around 8 p.m., skipping the nightcap.

10.4

The most important factor to watch out for is late-night junk food, which many of us are accused of (especially occasionally).

Dr. Longo's recommendation is to avoid eating food within 3 to 4 hours of going to bed. Keep things easy yet vigilant: restrict your eating to a 12hrs span. If you begin at 9:00 am, for example, make sure you finish by 9:00 p.m.

10.5
Restrict portion size, not feeding window, to lose weight

To reduce weight, restrict your portion sizes rather than your eating window.

How can you get the amount mostly on the scale to shift if you're already limiting your foods to a 12-hrs window?

Dr. Longo recommends cutting back to 2 meals & a snack per day instead of his normal 3 meals & a pair of snacks.

Obese or overweight people are more inclined to overeat any time they feed, which is why reducing the amount of meals & snacks is important for those trying to lose weight.

Listen to what the body is asking you it's often important to pay attention to and understand the body. Overeating can occur if people feel constrained, according to mouse studies. Fasting on weekdays, though, seems to help inhibit weight gain in mice in another review. TRF isn't for you if it makes you feel more anxious and encourages you to add weight. There are a variety of other diets to follow, including the Mediterranean and low-carb diets.

Different criteria refer to different body shapes. Dr. Longo proposes the following, depending on his own study and experience:

- People looking to reduce weight — men with waist circumferences greater than 40 inches & women with waist circumferences greater than 34 inches — can enjoy breakfast, lunch, and dinner, as well as a healthful, low-sugar snack.
- Men with waist circumferences of less than 33 inches & women with circumferences of less than 27 inches can have three meals and two snacks a day.

From Dr. Longo's Book, here are some balanced meal ideas

- Whole-wheat focaccia and blueberry jam for breakfast (no sugar added)
- Spinach and pine nuts & raisins for lunch
- Pasta, broccoli & black beans for dinner
- Snack: carrots, a handful of nuts, or a bar of dark chocolate

Dr. Longo's advice: It's important to keep portion sizes under control at all times. Rather than measuring calories, check food labeling to see if you're receiving enough calcium, minerals, omega fatty acids, and vitamins.

10.6 Don't skip to have breakfast

It's normal for us to miss breakfast and wait until 1:00 p.m. to consume their 1st meal, but Dr. Longo firmly recommends against it.

Although no precise link has been established, reports show that people who miss breakfast have significantly higher rates of cardiovascular disease, cancer, and death. They're much most likely to have poor cardiovascular and physical wellbeing.

If you do miss a meal, allow this lunch or dinner, & avoid snacking until bedtime.

Although Dr. Longo agrees that there are other possible reasons for why missing breakfast is linked to an elevated risk of mortality, he believes that this connection alone could be cause for alarm.

As per Dr. Longo, there is relatively little harmful evidence correlated with 12-hrs TRF, which is utilized for the majority of long-lived communities around the world.

Breakfast doesn't have to be a pain, according to Dr. Longo. If you normally eat late in the day owing to time restrictions or necessity, coffee or small breakfast of tea and toast with preserves will easily be integrated into the ones morning routine.

There is no fast track to wellness

Since there is no easy cure for perfect health, TRF isn't a quick fix for great health.

This way of eating could not be suitable for everyone's lifestyle. Fasting will not be for you whether it encourages you to drink or overeat on cheat days or weekends. (Harvard Health reports that 38% of those who attempted fasting gave up.)

If you're worried of TRF, speaking to the doctor first. For those with such illnesses, such as asthma, or others who have a history of disturbing feeding, missing meals, and reducing calorie consumption is not advised.

Making small, gradual changes to your lifestyle is the key to living life to the fullest. An easy fix isn't the solution like it isn't for healthier eating plans. It's just about laying a strong base for your long-term wellbeing.

10.7 What would you drink without breaking ones fast during intermittent fasting?

An RD describes which drinks are safe to consume & which can be avoided.

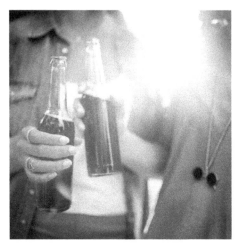

Intermittent fasting, a form of eating that's sometimes correlated to highprotein or ketogenic diets, poses a number of concerns, particularly if you're unfamiliar with it. You may be asking what kind of fasting schedule to try, what the legitimate health advantages are, whether you'll get any side effects, & what kind of weight-loss outcomes you might achieve. Another popular issue is whether you should drink drinks such as coffee or water when fasting.

The simple response is that it depends on the liquid you're consuming and the sort of IF diet you're on. However, according to New Jersey-based nutritionist Erin Palinski-Wade, RD, writer of 2 Day Diabetes Diet, "a safe rule of thumb is to skip certain beverages that contain any calories when you're fasting."

When you're attempting to sustain a fasted state, eating certain sugars, proteins, or fats will counteract the weight-loss effects from intermittent fasting, she notes. IF diets are often believed to better regulate blood sugar and reduce insulin resistance, all of which will lower the risk of being diabetic. If you eat so many liquid calories during what may be a fasted state, these advantages can be easily negated.

10.8 Award-winning fitness options from Women's Health

Here's what you need to know about some of the more common beverages you may want to drink when doing intermittent fasting, as well as whether or not they'll break your fast.

Coffee

You should drink it straight up. Since black coffee has no calories, it's fine to drink during a quick. Using cream, sugar, or milk, on the other hand, is better avoided since it adds calories to the drink, and will cause you to lose your fasting condition.

"Experiment with calorie-free flavoring from a spice like cinnamon if you do want to flavor your coffee during a fast," Palinski-Wade suggests. "Save the coffee incorporate for when you're not in a rush."

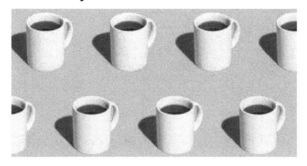

Is Caffeine Ideal For Weight Reduction Or Bad For It?

If you're fasting, limit yourself to one cup of coffee or turn to decaf. She believes that too much caffeine, particularly on an empty stomach, can create jittery feelings, which can increase appetite & the need to snack.

Tea

Take a chance. Tea, like coffee, is naturally calorie-free and appropriate to consume during a fast whether it is merely brewed tea made from leaves, tea bags, or flakes. If you want to drink ice tea from a cup, make sure it's unsweetened and clear of artificial sugar & calories, recommends Palinski-Wade. Caloric additions such as sugar, tea, or cream, like chocolate, can be saved for non-fasting hours.

"Because tea is usually lower in caffeine as compare to coffee, you may have a little more during fasts," she notes, noting that she likes decaf wherever possible.

Seltzer & water

Take a sip. According to Palinski-Wade, water is actually calorie-free, so there's no reason to limit it. Water is a healthy thing to drink during fasting periods not only to stay hydrated but also to fill the stomach and avoid hunger.

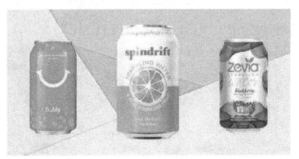

If you like flavored water, Palinski-Wade recommends adding fruit wedges or lime juice or a splash of lemon(or a juice) as long as it's a real "splash" (around 1 tbsp. per 12 ounces) & doesn't contain more than a few calories. As long as the carbonated drink/seltzer is naturally flavored & calorie-free, it may be viewed similarly to water.

Soda

It's best to avoid it. If you're curious if you should drink soda (or soda) when doing intermittent fasting, Dr. Palinski-Wade suggests avoiding soda in general, particularly if you're not on an intermittent fasting diet.

She claims that regular sodas are normally high in sugar & calories and have a little health benefit. There isn't enough evidence or study to tell if diet soda is safe to consume during whether, but studies show that drinking so much artificial sweeteners (which diet sodas typically contain) will enhance cravings & appetite, as well as encourage weight gain and fat accumulation.

"The safest choice is to drink as less soda as possible and ease the carbonated water or carbonation cravings with seltzer," she advises.

Alcohol

Don't mess about it. According to Palinski-Wade, alcohol can never be eaten after a fasting time since the symptoms are exacerbated when taken on an empty stomach. Alcohol is a calorie-dense liquor, but consuming it will break your fast whilst still enhancing your appetite & rising desire and cravings.

10.9 What about getting vitamins when you're fasting?

This is contingent on your fasting schedule, and you can contact the doctor before starting any supplements, according to Palinski-Wade. If you pace for a certain number of hours per day, take your vitamins at that period (unless a dietitian or doctor advises you otherwise), since certain nutrients, such as a multivitamin, are best absorbed when consumed with food.

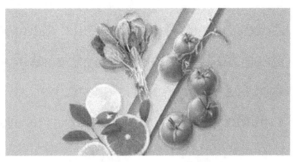

Vitamin-Rich Foods to Include in Your Diet

Supplements are still recommended if you observe extended fasting, which includes fasting on particular days, such as the 5:2 diet, to ensure you are fulfilling your food requirements per day. When pursuing every IF strategy, Palinski-Wade suggests taking a high-quality multivitamin every day.

"A fast day will not be compensated by the tiny number of calories contained in a gummy/chewable/liquid vitamin," she notes. "However, contact the doctor or dietitian first to guarantee that you will take one's supplement on an empty stomach."

Chapter 11: OMAD Diet

This chapter is all about the one meal a day diet. From studies and researches, we have come to the conclusion is that this is the form of diet people tend to follow more, some deliberate and some undeliberate. You will know everything about this diet in detail over here. You will get to know all the conditions in which he knows when one should plan to start this diet and when someone should avoid this diet. Let us begin with the details that what would really happen if you attempt this diet.

11.1
What happens when we attempt extreme fasting by just eating once a day?

You might lose weight by eating pizza & burgers a day and drinking beer, but is that a smart idea?

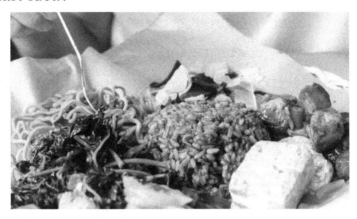

When you first began looking into the 1 Meal a Day Diet (OMAD), it was the plan's simplicity that may draw you in: you consume one meal a day, consists of what you'd like, usually at dinnertime.

Super unconventional, right?

The OMAD, on the other hand, is essentially a more intense cousin or an extreme form of intermittent fasting of the Warrior Diet. OMAD differs from conventional fasting in that rather than fasting for the average window of 16 hrs. you fast for around 23 hrs. (Including that time also you spend sleeping).

If the idea seems a bit shady, like a mid-infomercial hawking a nutritional aid, let's look at the logic — and research — from all sides of the argument before dismissing it completely.

Why eat only once per day?

The possibility of skipping a single meal making several people squirm. Any day, deliberately skipping all but 1 meal appears wasteful and needless. However, supporters of OMAD assert a slew of advantages, including:

● **Improved concentration & output.** Who hasn't witnessed the groggy 2:30 pm. slump at work? Since there is no lunch, OMAD is said to eradicate the sluggishness people experience when digesting their meal. ● **Loss of weight**. When you only consume once a day, it's difficult to be in caloric excess. Even if your 1 meal isn't "good" by popular means, you're not consuming nearly as many calories as if you fed during the day.

● **Dietary freedom.** Forget of calorie counting and dining out of the cool box. When you don't have to prepare four to 6 meals a day, you open a lot of mental resources.

Any people feed in this manner for religious purposes. Others, such as former athletes Ronda Rousey & Herschel Walker, tend to feed just once each day for the remainder of their lives. Walker appears to have been consuming just one meal a day for years, normally a salad and bread in the evening.

Before the middle Ages, there is also empirical proof that the Romans only consumed one big meal a day.

Our first experience with OMAD

We fed once a day several times during my OMAD experimentation, but never for a prolonged period of time. The longest streak we ever had was five days. We've carried weights, practiced full-court hoops, and done several forms of strenuous workout whilst fasted on many occasions.

Below are the top three takeaways from playing with the OMAD diet:

1. Just but you have the desire to eat something doesn't mean you do.

We got swept up in the childish glee of being allowed to consume anything we wanted early on in our OMAD eating.

11.3

Then we remembered we had just eaten wings, nachos, and whisky in the preceding 48 hrs. This is unquestionably not the best fuel for a balanced body.

Yes, part of the charm of OMAD is the freedom to consume anything you want, but for the sake of your better wellbeing, you can try to keep your one meal healthy & micronutrient rich.

2. It is unlikely to be suitable for intense strength exercise.

We are a regular lifter. On OMAD, we didn't find any significant lack of power, but we weren't really hammering the iron either.

Restricting one's meals won't help him if he is just lifting for overall health & not for results.

Severe lifters, on the other hand, who wish to improve their intensity over time want to try a less drastic form of OMAD, such as a standard 16:8 feeding window or the Warrior Diet.

3. It's a perfect way to boost your willpower and discipline.

One of the motives you pursued OMAD is to see whether you had the moral fortitude to avoid food. It might be difficult because hunger is a strong emotion. You might gave in & had lunch for several days.

Still, for the most part, you will be satisfied with yourself for keeping to the diet & felt free to indulge yourself with a hearty lunch. If you agree that consistency is a muscle that needs to be improved, OMAD is one solution to consider, one that will help you stay in better shape.

11.4 What does research tell about the advantages and drawbacks of OMAD?

Just because a lot of people do stuff doesn't mean it's right for you. When it comes to whether or not it's healthy to consume just one meal a day, the data is mixed.

According to a 2007 survey, feeding only once a day raises blood pressure & cholesterol. So, even though you're gaining weight, if your 1 meal per day consists of too much plain carbohydrates, or heavily refined fried foods you'll feel pretty terrible.

- Fasting can also face the following risks: a
- heavy urge to eating or excessive feeding
- physical weakness or trembling low energy
- or fatigue
- Fog in the head, or inability to concentrate

However, a small 2017 study of 10 persons with type 2 diabetes found that fasting for 18-20 hrs. a day can contribute to better blood glucose control.

If one has diabetes, though, long-term OMAD is definitely not for you. Of necessity, before undertaking any big lifestyle adjustments, you can contact a doctor.

Fasting can increase the body's resilience to disease by placing cells under "healthy tension," similar to how lifting weights produces tears that allow muscle fibers to develop back stronger, according to research published in 2005.

In a 2016 trial with mice, longer fasts with just water consumed were related to a lower risk of diseases including cancer & diabetes.

Limited, liquid fasts did not result in either long-term medical risks, according to a 2018 chart review of 768 medical-facility patients.

Most stable adults are possibly safe to quick every now and then, according to the medical opinion. The studies listed here, on the other hand, relate to days of water-only fasting or general intermittent fasting. There isn't a lot of research on the dangers and advantages of OMAD.

Chapter 12: 10 Popular Mistakes to Avoid During Intermittent Fasting

When it comes to intermittent fasting, there are 10 popular Mistakes to avoid.

It can seem that skipping meals and reducing caloric consumption is easy but read on before embarking on an intermittent fast.

Intermittent fasting is a practice of eating under which you alternate between eating and fasting times. "Intermittent fasting may be part of a healthier lifestyle," according to Johns Hopkins who has researched the health effects of intermittent fasting for 25 years and embraced it himself around 20 years ago. According to him, evidence shows that minimizing your "eating time" will help you live longer and reduce your threat of chronic diseases.

12.1 Ten popular mistakes while fasting

Do you think you up for a sporadic fast? While spacing out meals & snacks seems to be an easy task, you can easily destroy your quick if you make these mistakes. **1. You do not ease in it.**

Breakfast is optional. Lunch may be skipped. You are willing to feed your arm by 3:00 pm As per Libby Mills, RD, who is a dietitian "if you usually eat every 3 4 hours and then immediately shrink your feeding cycle to an 8hour span, you'll definitely feel constantly hungry & discouraged."

"Weight reduction can be a motivator for limiting the eating hours. This, on the other hand, is a chance to reconnect with the body's true feelings. We feed every 3-4 hours on average, & not always as we are starving." Plus, you won't have to fast for the whole week. In reality, people who observe the 5:2 diet consume a daily amount of nutritious food for five days and reduce their calorie consumption for the remaining two days. People who reduced calories twice regularly lost a significant amount as anyone who limited calories constantly, according to a survey involving 107 obese or overweight women.

2. You're consuming too Much Calories.

According to Mills, you're not alone. "It's convenient to overeat after a quick end, either because you are hungry or because you convince yourself that you compensating for the calories you've missed." She proposes using a 0-10 scale, with 0 suggesting starvation & 10 indicating fullness. You must be hungry before eating & avoid eating until you're fulfilled, not just to finish your plate. She also advises feeding steadily so the brain has ample time to indicate that you're finished. "After you start feeding, it might take 15 to 20 minutes," Mills says.

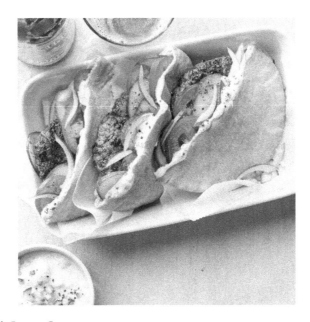

3. You destroy with soda

According to Mills, the carbonation of soda will disguise your appetite, setting you up by being too hungry during your next meal & leading to overeating. "Artificially sweetened beverages will even increase the pleasure bar for sweet tastes, but a slice of fruit cannot be enjoyable when you do consume it." (Learn more about chemical sweeteners and their effects on the body.)

She also mentions that these drinks can contain caffeine, which has varying effects on various individuals. "Caffeine can make you feel jittery & make you crave candy. Other sources of caffeine, on the other hand, can mask your hunger and cause you to delay eating until you are no longer hungry."

4. You're not keeping track of how much water you're consuming.

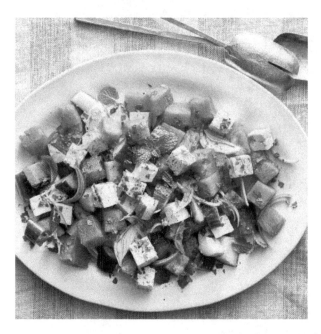

In general, 2 liters (half a gallon) of water should be consumed every day "Water is a component of our body's metabolic reactions and is needed for it to work properly. We can't confuse hunger with thirst if we're well-hydrated "Mills makes a point.

At snack breaks, pick non-starchy, water-rich vegetables and fruits (yes, hydrating foods count against your regular water goal.). Prepare celery, sliced cucumbers, watermelon, and oranges in advance and store them in the refrigerator or in a lunch bag.

5. You're not breaking the fast with the right foods.

According to Mills, consuming enough lean protein (meat, poultry, plantbased proteins & seafood,), nuts, & seeds with each meal can help you stay fuller for longer. "Protein makes one feel satisfied. Protein can also help you preserve your metabolically healthy lean body mass if you're missing a few pounds."

Another advantage, according to Mills, is that fiber from fruits, veggies, whole grains, and legumes slows the processing and absorption of carbohydrates, keeping you satisfied and energized longer b/w meals. "Plus, eating foods that include nutrition and fiber would provide you with the minerals, vitamins, and nutrients you'll need when you re-portion calorie intake," she says.

6. The approach is unnecessarily zealous.

Sure, you want to snatch this diet craze by the lapels & fly with it, but you don't have to go hungry. If you consume fewer than 800 calories a day, you'll lose more weight (and have a lot more hunger), but you'll lose more bone mass. In the long run, it isn't safe or viable. Not to mention that if you find your window of not consuming too lengthy, you would be unable to maintain it. Smaller, more manageable modifications can be made, and you should still listen to your body.

7. You are suffering from caffeine withdrawal

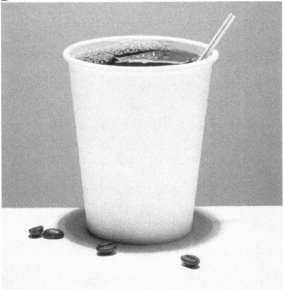

Who says you couldn't get a cup of coffee in the morning, an espresso in the afternoon, or a cup of hot tea in the evening? Nobody. In reality, coffee isn't harmful to your health. "A caffeinated beverage, particularly if it's hot," Mills says, "is a soothing bridge b/w meals." If you're fasting, remember not to add milk or sugar to your cup.

8. You are In Your Own Head

Intermittent fasting can seem like a normal part of your schedule, whether you do it for a week or a month. "It makes sense over a lifetime to shift the emphasis to become more intuitive on what you feed depending on your sensations of hunger & fullness," Mills says.

"Choosing foods that supply the body with nutrients it takes to remain energized moves your attitude from calorie counting to quality of life." It's more like a modern way of thinking about—& consuming—food than a diet.

9. You partake in a strenuous, high-intensity exercise.

You should exercise, but not in the same manner as the Hulk. When the tank is low, it's difficult to go full out in a workout. Moderate activity is beneficial to your fitness, so if you'd rather be a bit more intense, make sure you are not hungry for hours. Basically, do go to the gym until 5 a.m. and don't eat before 2 p.m. To bring you through a difficult workout & replenish your stocks afterward, your body requires gasoline.

10. You give up since you ate at the wrong time.

Don't give up & don't be too hard on yourself. You won't lose all your hard work with a single meal, but a poor attitude could. Take some time to reassess to make sure the routine you've developed is still working for you. Maybe it does not anymore, and you'd want to change or relax you are eating window. That's fine. Care to pay attention to your dietary preferences and consume high-quality, healthy items as practicable. You would not be hungry all day if you consume a healthy diet of protein, fiber, non-starchy vegetables, and water.

According to a Scientist, these are the Safest Vegetables for Gut well-being. They Are the Most Delicious Vegetables.

Conclusion

Intermittent fasting is a weight-loss strategy that works for certain individuals but not for others.

Some claim that it might not be as helpful to women as it is to men. It's still not a safe thing for individuals who have or are at risk of having an eating disorder.

Being a woman when you plan to attempt intermittent fasting, note that the consistency of your food is important. It's impossible to hope to lose weight & improve your fitness by bingeing on fast food at mealtimes. While several interesting results have been discovered, the implications of intermittent fasting in metabolism are being researched.

Humans have evolved to be able to fast from time to time. It has been shown in recent studies to be beneficial for weight reduction, metabolic fitness, cancer prevention, and perhaps also helping you live longer. Early evidence in women over the age of 50 shows that short-term fasts will increase metabolism by up to 14%, and some reports show that intermittent fasting does not lead to significant muscle loss.

If this is the case, intermittent fasting has a number of significant weightloss benefits over diets dependent on calorie restriction. Bear in mind that if you want to add lean muscle & reduce weight, you'll need to keep track of your body fat. Don't look at the scale and see how you're making strides. It is deceptive.

Learn how intermittent fasting will help you lose weight by allowing you to liquefy fat without relying on food, drink, or exercise. Understand how converting to a one-morning routine will help you burn fat quicker than any other process.

Discover the most successful diet to mix with intermittent fasting to energize the "great" creatures in your stomach to fulfill their "housekeeping duties" & keep your body safe.

Get the most important weight loss without being hungry or getting drained... (You will definitely feel more motivated than you do in the past.) How to use this technique to reverse physical aging... and keep the lines at bay.

How to still use this approach to cure age-related illnesses & increase the average lifespan by at least 30 percent. Explore how intermittent fasting changes your proclivities to your science, helping you to focus on mending rather than crushing your body.

Comprehend how intermittent fasting softens fat stores by allowing you to eat nutrition 14 percent faster. Study how intermittent fasting affects the "weight-gain" hormone of yours & reduces your chances of developing stoutness, coronary artery disease, type 2 diabetes, and malignant growth.

Learn how intermittent fasting causes a concoction that slashes the muscleto-fat ratio like such a jack-hammer into wood. Learn how intermittent fasting produces a torpid object that concocts your bulk by knowing the theory behind it (without the requirement of activity)

Learn how a particular intermittent fasting strategy boosts your metabolism, which increases the rate of fat copying due to the increased demand on the body (this is rather to be appreciative for)

Study how a particular intermittent fasting method washes down the stomach, helping you to absorb & ingest nourishment into your circulation system with better performance.

Finally, for women, intermittent fasting may be a particularly useful weight loss technique. Intermittent fasting can also help to delay the aging process by reducing weight, blood pressure, and cholesterol, according to a Harvard report.

Is intermittent fasting, then, potentially beneficial? Are there any advantages? Are there any pitfalls? Read this book to have all your burning questions addressed before determining whether it's correct for you or not.

If you have read the book till the end you are very much familiar now with what is intermittent fasting and how it should be followed. Remember one thing before beginning your venture on this beautiful journey of weight loss by intermittent fasting that you don't have to rush, penitence is the key here.

Another important thing which one should keep in mind is that this book is specially made for elderly women (over the age of 50), who still want them to look young, healthy, fit, beautiful and attractive. So the basic guidelines are for this age group of the specific gender and one should be careful regarding the dos and don'ts of intermittent fasting.

We hope you will have a good time reading it as no stone is left unturned in writing this book for your better understanding and easy guidance. We wish you the best of luck and hope that you may find this book in the best of your interest.